Dr. C. A. Young
The Walton Centre for
Neurology and Neurosurgery

Physical Medicine and Rehabilitation

Outcome Measurement

Guest Editor:

Richard M. Smith, PhD

Senior Research Scientist
Rehabilitation Foundation, Inc.
Wheaton, Illinois

Volume 11/Number 2 June 1997
HANLEY & BELFUS, INC. Philadelphia

STATE OF THE ART REVIEWS

Publisher: HANLEY & BELFUS, INC.
210 South 13th Street
Philadelphia, PA 19107
(215) 546-7293
(215) 790-9330 (Fax)
Web site: http://www.hanleyandbelfus.com

This volume is based upon papers presented at the First International Outcome Measurement Conference, co-sponsored by Rehabilitation Foundation, Inc., and the MESA Psychometric Laboratory at the University of Chicago, May 31–June 1, 1996, Chicago, IL.

The Second International Outcome Measurement Conference will be held May 15–16, 1998, at the International House, University of Chicago, 1414 East 59th Street, Chicago, IL 60637. For further information, please contact:

Richard M. Smith, PhD
Rehabilitation Foundation, Inc.
26W171 Roosevelt Road
PO Box 675
Wheaton, IL 60189

Phone: 630-462-4102
Fax: 630-462-4547
E-mail: jomea@rfi.org

PHYSICAL MEDICINE AND REHABILITATION: State of the Art Reviews is included in *BioSciences Information Service, Current Contents, ISI/BIOMED,* and *Cumulative Index to Nursing & Allied Health Literature.*

PHYSICAL MEDICINE AND REHABILITATION: State of the Art Reviews ISSN 0888-7357
Volume 11, Number 2 ISBN 1-56053-234-3

PHYSICAL MEDICINE AND REHABILITATION: State of the Art Reviews is published triannually (three times per year) by Hanley & Belfus, Inc., 210 South 13th Street, Philadelphia, Pennsylvania 19107.

POSTMASTER: Send address changes to PHYSICAL MEDICINE AND REHABILITATION: State of the Art Reviews, Hanley & Belfus, Inc., 210 South 13th Street, Philadelphia, PA 19107.

Physical Medicine and Rehabilitation: State of the Art Reviews
Vol. 11, No. 2, June 1997

OUTCOME MEASUREMENT
Richard M. Smith, PhD

CONTENTS

1995 ISSUES

Rehabilitation of Fractures
Arun J. Mehta, MB, Editor
Sepulveda, California

Sexuality and Disability
Trilok N. Monga, MD, Editor
Houston, Texas

Spinal Rehabilitation
Mark A. Young, MD, and
Robert A. Lavin, MD, Editors
Baltimore, Maryland

1996 ISSUES

The Autonomic Nervous System
Robert W. Teasell, MD, Editor
London, Ontario, Canada

Sympathetic Pain Syndromes:
Reflex Sympathetic Dystrophy and Causalgia
C. David Tollison, PhD, and
John R. Satterthwaite, MD, Editors
Greenville, South Carolina

Physiatric Anatomic Principles
Kamala Shankar, MD, Editor
Stanford, California

1997 ISSUES

Advances in Rehabilitation Technology
Trilok N. Monga, MD, and Kuno P. Zimmermann, DO, PhD, Editors
Houston, Texas

Outcome Measurement
Richard M. Smith, PhD, Editor

Functional Biomechanics and Rehabilitation of Sports Injuries
Joseph D. Fortin, DO, Frank Falco, MD, and
Hilaire A.C. Jacob, PhD, Editors
Fort Wayne, Indiana; Wilmington, Delaware; and Zurich, Switzerland

Subscriptions for full year and single issues available from the publisher—
Hanley & Belfus, Inc., 210 South 13th Street, Philadelphia, PA 19107.
Telephone (215) 546-7293; (800) 962-1892. Fax (215) 790-9330.

CONTRIBUTORS

Richard F. Averill, MS
Research Manager, 3M Health Information Systems, Wallingford, Connecticut

John G. Baker, PhD
Clinical Assistant Professor, Department of Rehabilitation Medicine (CFAR), State University of New York at Buffalo, Buffalo, New York

Rita K. Bode, PhD
Post-Doctoral Fellow, Rehabilitation Institute of Chicago, Chicago, Illinois

David Cella, PhD
Department of Psychology, Rush Presbyterian-St. Luke's Medical Center, Chicago, Illinois

Chih-Hung Chang, PhD
Department of Psychology, Rush Presbyterian-St. Luke's Medical Center, Chicago, Illinois

Herbert Fillmore, MA
Director of Research, Village Comprehensive Care, New York, New York

Anne G. Fisher, ScD, OTR, FAOTA
Professor, Department of Occupational Therapy, Colorado State University, Fort Collins, Colorado

William P. Fisher, Jr., PhD
Associate Professor, Department of Public Health and Preventive Medicine, Louisiana State University Medical Center, New Orleans, Louisiana

Norbert I. Goldfield, MD
Director, 3M Health Information Systems, Wallingford, Connecticut

Carl V. Granger, MD
Professor, Department of Rehabilitation Medicine; Director, CFAR/UDSMR, Rehabilitation Medicine, State University of New York at Buffalo, Buffalo, New York

Thelma Grant, MBA, RRA
Senior Product Development Analyst, 3M Health Information Systems, Wallingford, Connecticut

Dennis J. Graziano, BBA
Program Manager, New York State Department of Health, New York, New York

Allen W. Heinemann, PhD
Professor, Department of Physical Medicine and Rehabilitation, Northwestern University Medical School, Rehabilitation Institute of Chicago, Chicago, Illinois

Jin-Shei Lai, PhD, OTR/L
Research Assistant Professor, Department of Occupational Therapy, University of Illinois at Chicago, Chicago, Illinois

John Michael Linacre, PhD
Associate Director, MESA Psychometric Laboratory, University of Chicago, Chicago, Illinois

Rodney Richard Schall, PhD
Director, Department of Psychology, Good Shepherd Rehabilitation Hospital, Allentown, Pennsylvania

Mary Segal, PhD
Assistant Professor, Department of Physical Medicine and Rehabilitation, Temple University School of Medicine; Research Scientist, Moss Rehabilitation Research Institute, Moss Rehabilitation Hospital, Philadelphia, Pennsylvania

Richard M. Smith, PhD
Senior Research Scientist, Rehabilitation Foundation Inc., Wheaton, Illinois

Alan Tennant, BA
Charterhouse Principal Research Fellow, Rheumatology and Rehabilitation Research Unit, University of Leeds, Leeds, United Kingdom

Craig A. Velozo, PhD, OTR
Associate Professor, Department of Occupational Therapy, University of Illinois at Chicago, Chicago, Illinois

Yvette Wang, MS
Advanced Software Engineer, 3M Health Information Systems, Wallingford, Connecticut

Benjamin D. Wright, PhD
Professor of Psychology and Education, Director MESA Psychometric Laboratory, University of Chicago, Chicago, Illinois

C. Young, MD
The Walton Center for Neurology and Neurosurgery, Liverpool, United Kingdom

PREFACE

The articles in this volume are based on papers presented at the First International Outcome Measurement Conference, co-sponsored by Rehabilitation Foundation, Inc., and the MESA Psychometric Laboratory at the University of Chicago. The conference was the first of a biennial series of meetings designed to bring together practitioners of outcome measurement in the health sciences. This conference focused on outcome measurement in physical medicine and rehabilitation. Outcome measurement has been an important topic for PM&R since the mid-1980s. The articles in this volume highlight some of the scales (PECS, FIM, and Barthel) that have pioneered the use of Rasch measurement models in this field. The theme of this volume is transcending individual scales in PM&R and working toward developing a common metric.

Throughout the development of scientific knowledge in this area there have been several common threads that can be identified. The first is the development of interval scales to change the ordinal observations on which most data are based into measures that are amenable to the types of statistical analysis usually used with these types of data. The second is the standardization of all of the competing interval scales into a common metric that allows practitioners to communicate in a common language. These two steps are usually precursors to substantial increases in the theoretical and practical knowledge about a given field of inquiry. The Rasch measurement models used in all of these papers provide the capacity to accomplish these two steps. The first step has been accomplished and is well documented in this volume. The field of PM&R is just beginning to recognize the importance of the second step. Several of the articles in this volume illustrate initial phases of accomplishing this goal.

The first chapter, by Benjamin D. Wright, details the rationale of developing linear unidimensional scales with the family of Rasch psychometric models. The next six chapters provide an overview of various applications of these models. Anne Fisher details the development of an ADL scale based on the FACETS models that includes measurement of the rater parameter. The Baker and Granger chapter details the development of a follow-along tool that supplements the FIM, a commonly used outcome tool for inpatient rehabilitation outcomes. The Linacre chapter provides insight into how the common metric for persons and items developed from the FIM can be used to its fullest advantage in developing self-scoring forms that allow clinicians immediate feedback on person measures and the internal consistency of the item scores that underlie the measure. The Lai, Velozo, and Linacre chapter illustrates how the FACETS model can be used to investigate the variability in rater severity across a national data base. This work also uses the FIM as a means of demonstrating how this problem can be investigated and controlled. The Smith chapter is the last of the chapters on applications for single scales. This chapter explores the common structure of the metrics developed from the use of PECS as both a status evaluation and a goal-setting scale. The Goldfield chapter demonstrates how linear unidimensional scales can be used in improving prediction of outcomes.

The chapter by William Fisher is the first of a group of papers that relate to the development of scale-free measurement scales for functional outcomes. This chapter provides the theoretical basis for combining different outcome scales into a single common metric that can be used to compare outcomes regardless of the outcome scale used in the assessment. The Tennant and Young chapter is the first of the practical examples, showing how the Barthel and the physical medicine section of the SF-36 were co-calibrated. The Segal and Heinemann chapter provides the details of the co-calibration of the FIM and the SF-36. Both of these papers are examples of the process that William Fisher describes for developing a common metric for functional outcome scales. The Cella and Chang chapter uses the same methodology but applies it to health status instruments used in an applied oncology setting. This methodology can be applied to different instruments or to the same instrument translated into several languages.

In the final chapter, Bode and Heinemann look at completion of the FIM by different clinicians. These results suggest that there may be different definitions of the variable depending on the clinical area represented by the person completing the evaluation.

We hope that you will find these chapters interesting and informative. They represent important steps in achieving what William Fisher describes as the "Gold Standard" for measuring functional outcomes.

Richard M. Smith, PhD
GUEST EDITOR

PUBLISHED ISSUES 1987–1994

(available from the publisher)

August 1987
Medical Complications of Spinal Cord Injury
Mark N. Ozer, MA, and
James K. Schmitt, MD, Editors

February 1988
Joint, Soft Tissue, and Disk Disorders
Robert L. Swezey, MD, Editor

May 1988
Rehabilitation of the Alcoholic
Curtis Wright, MD, Editor

August 1988
Home Health Care and Rehabilitation
Jay Portnow, MD, PhD, Editor

November 1988
Rehabilitation of Neuromuscular Diseases
William M. Fowler, Jr., MD, Editor

February 1989
Traumatic Brain Injury
Lawrence J. Horn, MD, and
D. Nathan Cope, MD, Editors

May 1989
Quantifying Neurologic Performance
Ross Davis, MD, George V. Kondraske, PhD,
Wallace W. Tourtellotte, MD, PhD, and
Karl Syndulko, PhD, Editors

August 1989
Medical Management of the Elderly Stroke Patient
Roy V. Erickson, MD, Editor

November 1989
Clinical Electrophysiology
Daniel Dumitru, MD, Editor

February 1990
Rehabilitation of the Aging Population
F. Patrick Maloney, MD, and
Kevin M. Means, MD, Editors

June 1990
Neck and Back Pain
Jeffrey A. Saal, MD, Editor

October 1990
The Coma-Emerging Patient
Elizabeth Sandel, MD, and
David W. Ellis, PhD, Editors

February 1991
Rehabilitation of Chronic Pain
Nicolas E. Walsh, MD, Editor

June 1991
The Child with Physical Disability
Gabriella Molnar, MD, Editor

October 1991
Musculoskeletal Pain
Constance D. Schwab, MD, Editor

February 1992
Post-Concussive Disorders
Lawrence J. Horn, MD, and
Nathan D. Zasler, MD, Editors

June 1992
Industrial Rehabilitation
Chrisanne Gordon, MD, and
Paul E. Kaplan, MD, Editors

October 1992
Neuropsychological Assessment
Stephanie Hanson, PhD, and
David Tucker, PhD, Editors

February 1993
Long-Term Consequences of Stroke
Robert W. Teasell, MD, Editor

June 1993
Management for Rehabilitation Medicine II
F. Patrick Maloney, MD, and
Richard P. Gray, MD, Editors

September 1993
HIV-Related Disability: Assessment and Management
Michael W. O'Dell, MD, Editor

October 1993
Neurologic and Orthopaedic Sequelae of Traumatic Brain Injury
Lance R. Stone, DO, Editor

February 1994
Prosthetics
Alberto Esquenazi, MD, Editor

June 1994
Cancer Rehabilitation
Fae H. Garden, MD, and
Martin Grabois, MD, Editors

October 1994
Spasticity
Richard T. Katz, MD, Editor

BENJAMIN D. WRIGHT, PHD

FUNDAMENTAL MEASUREMENT FOR OUTCOME EVALUATION

From the MESA Psychometric Laboratory
University of Chicago
Chicago, Illinois

Reprint requests to:
Benjamin D. Wright, PhD
MESA
5835 Kimbark
Chicago, IL 60637

All measures are numbers, but not all numbers are measures. Some numbers, such as those on car licenses, are merely labels. Others, such as room numbers, name a location. The number may help us to find the room, but it does not tell us how many steps it takes to get there.

Other numbers are provided as counts, scores, and ranks: 10 hospital days, 17 rating scale points, and third place. Because these numbers are obtained by direct observation, they have the reality of being seen to occur. As a result, these kinds of numbers are often mistaken for measures and misused in statistical analyses for which they are quite unsuited.

Counts, scores, and ranks do not qualify as measurements because the "reality" of these concrete units guarantees that their relevance to our reason for counting them cannot be uniform. Some "days" are worth more than others. How far is it from first to second place?

Finally, there are the numbers that deserve to be called measures. These are counts of abstract generic units, such as dollars, degrees and pounds. Each unit is a perfect idea that can only be approximated in practice. But its good-enough-for-practice approximation is what produces the kind of numbers that make the work of physical scientists, engineers, architects, businessmen, tailors, and cooks useful and productive. Genuine "measures" and not mere "scores" are the kind of numbers we need to evaluate outcomes.

When we use numbers to compare outcomes, we do arithmetic with them. We add and divide to compute means. We subtract to compare alternatives and gauge improvements. We calculate rates of change to estimate costs and weigh the effects of exposure and treatment.

Arithmetic done with numerical labels makes nonsense, and arithmetic done with counts, scores, and ranks also can be misleading. We must learn how to transcend this problem by the routine application of a simple mathematical model that constructs abstract linear measures from the concrete raw data for which counts, scores, and ranks are the media. For the arithmetic of statistical analysis to be useful, it must be done with equal interval, constant unit, linear measures. Nothing else will do.

WHICH NUMBERS ARE MEASURES?

How can we distinguish between numbers that are measures and numbers that are not? Measures are the kind of numbers that cooperate with arithmetic; they can be added, subtracted, multiplied, and divided. No one using numbers as labels, such as those on license plates, would do arithmetic with them. However, arithmetic is often attempted with numbers that are counts, scores, and ranks. Ratings mark out an order of increase. There is usually little doubt that a rating of two is meant to mean more than a rating of one and less than a rating of three. However, from the point of view of arithmetic, the questions unanswered by ratings are: How much more? How much less?

We may be able to believe in the rank order of ratings. Indeed, the best of incoming raw data is no more than ratings. But to be realistic, we have to admit that our ideas about the spacing between ratings are vague. We may feel sure that a rating of two is more than a rating of one. But we do not know how much more. Even though ratings specify order, they do not have the numerical properties necessary to serve arithmetic. Subtractions of ratings, sums of ratings, and, hence, averages and standard deviations of ratings are meaningless.

Another kind of observed number, the raw score, is often misused as though it were a measure because it is a count of what amount to ratings. But counting does not make raw scores any better for arithmetical analysis than the ratings themselves. When we add raw scores, we are counting "right" answers, but there is no reason to suppose that the right answers are all the same size. This realization is far from recent. In 1904 the founder of educational measurement, American psychologist Edward Thorndike, observed: "If one attempts to measure even so simple a thing as spelling, one is hampered by the fact that there exist no units in which to measure. One may arbitrarily make up a list of words and observe ability by the number spelled correctly. But if one examines such a list one is struck by the inequality of the units. All results based on the equality of any one word with any other are necessarily inaccurate."[28]

Thorndike saw the unavoidable ambiguity in counting concrete events, however indicative they might seem. One might observe signs of spelling ability, but one would not have measured spelling—at least not yet.[6–8] The problem of what to count, that is, entity ambiguity, is ubiquitous in science, commerce, and cooking. What is an apple? How many little apples make a big one? How rotten can an apple be and still get counted? Why don't three apples always cost the same amount? With apples, we solve entity ambiguity by renouncing the concrete apple count and turning, instead, to abstract apple volume or, better still, apple weight. This ambiguity as to the value of what is being counted makes raw scores unsuited to the arithmetic so mistakenly done with them.

What kind of numbers, then, are good enough to be subjected to arithmetic? Only numbers that approximate the idea of a perfectly uniform unit in which a difference of one between any two numbers always means exactly the same amount. Only then can we do arithmetic with the numbers. Only then can we make sense of means and standard deviations. Only then do we have numbers good enough to use as measures.

But these kinds of numbers do not occur naturally. Their perfection is only an abstraction. To obtain actual values for such numbers we must invent devices that produce good-enough approximations of our "perfect" units to be useful. The yardstick is the canonical example. We are content to use the inch marks on most yardsticks as though they were perfectly spaced at exactly one inch apart. However, the inch marks on any particular yardstick vary slightly in their spacing. Do we then abandon the yardstick? Absolutely not. All we require is that the inch-mark spacings approximate uniformity well enough to keep the yardstick useful as a device for measuring length, say to the nearest inch.

Many social scientists are confused about the difference between ratings, raw scores, and measures. They mistake ordinal ratings and scores for measures and attempt to understand their data by linear analyses of these ordinal values. Their results are inevitably ambiguous in arbitrary ways that remain unknown to them. Little wonder that there is so much confusion and contradiction and so little progress in contemporary social science. Outcome measurement cannot afford to suffer this mistake. The mistake is completely unnecessary. There is a simple, efficient, and easily applied method for constructing good approximations of abstract measures from concrete ordinal observations such as raw scores and ratings. This chapter discusses the unavoidable ambiguities in data collection; provides understanding of the ways in which raw scores and Likert scales are misleading when mistaken for measures; explains how raw, concrete observations such as ratings can be used to construct outcome measures; and gives some examples of the useful maps and scoring forms that follow from the construction of measures.

RATINGS

To measure treatment outcomes, we rate patients' typical functional independence on typical tasks of daily living according to scales such as the following:

1 – Maximally dependent
2 – Moderate assistance
3 – Minimal assistance
4 – Requires supervision
5 – Limited independence
6 – Functional independence
7 – Fully independent

When we use these ratings to evaluate a patient, we presume that we:

(a) Judge the patient correctly,
(b) According to reproducible criteria,
(c) With ratings accurately recorded,
(d) In terms of uniformly spaced levels like 1, 2, 3, 4, 5, 6, 7,
(e) Which add up to scores as good as measures.

But our presumptions are naive. Our ratings are no better than:

(a) Educated guesses,
(b) According to fluctuating personal criteria,
(c) Not always recorded correctly,
(d) In ordinal ratings,
(e) Which do not add up to measures.

RAW SCORES

Thorndike was not only aware of the "inequality of the units" but also of the nonlinearity of any resulting "raw scores." Raw scores are limited to begin at "none right" and to end at "all right." But the linear measures that we intend for raw scores to imply have no such bounds.

The monotonically increasing ogival exchange between raw scores and measures is illustrated in Figures 1 and 2. The horizontal x-axis in these figures is defined by linear measures. Their vertical y-axes are defined by raw score percents in Figure 1 and by raw score points in Figure 2.

The exchange of one more right answer for a measure increment is steepest where items are dense, usually toward the middle of a test near 50% right. At the extremes of 0% and 100% right, however, the exchange becomes flat. This means that for a symmetrical set of item difficulties, one more right answer implies the least measure increment near 50% but an infinite increment at each extreme.

Imagine a situation in which to measure a treatment outcome you inadvertently use a set of questions that are too easy to score, even before treatment. This unrealized mistargeting will make even the most effective treatment appear ineffective. The same will happen when the set of questions are too hard to score on. Indeed, the apparent effectiveness of the treatment in raw scores will depend entirely on how the questions are targeted on the sample of patients being examined. The size of the raw score increments produced by measure differences among patients and between treatments is entirely subject to the targeting of the test.

Figure 1 shows a typical raw score plotted against measure curve. This curve describes the nonlinear rating form raw score (in percent correct) to linear measure relationship of a functional ability measure. The horizontal measure distance between vertical scores of 88% and 98% is *five times* greater than the distance between scores of 45% and 55%, even though the raw score differences are an equivalent 10%.

Were we to evaluate the relative effectiveness of alternative treatments A and B in terms of their raw scores, with A centered at a measure of 0 logits and B centered

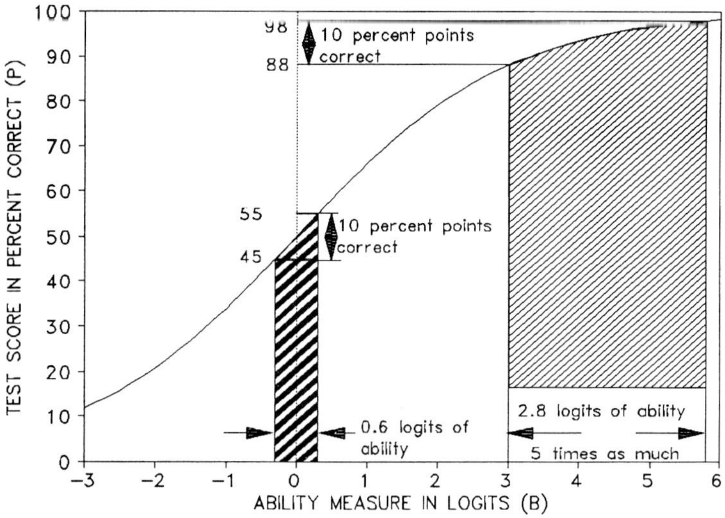

FIGURE 1. Extreme raw scores are biased against measures.

at 4.4 logits on the x-axis, we would be misled into concluding that the two treatments were equally effective even though the measures their scores imply show that treatment B is, in fact, five times more effective than treatment A.

Is there any way to confirm that the raw score bias ratio implied in Figure 1 is really five? To see that "five" is about right, imagine applying a new set of questions that measure along the same variable but are more difficult to score. Imagine the curve of this harder test to be similar in shape to the curve in Figure 1 but shifted 4.4 logits to the right so that it is centered on the 2.8 logit measure change of treatment B. When we use the new curve to look up the y-axis percent right intercepts for x-axis measures at 3 and 5.8 logits, they imply a raw score increase from 25% to 75% correct instead of 45% to 55%. This is a change of 50%, which is indeed five times greater than the previous change of 10%.

Thus, when we compare raw score changes by reexamining each change with a test centered on the region of that change, we get raw score ratios that resemble the measure ratios made explicit in Figure 1 for any change anywhere along any test. This shows how the linear measures, which can be constructed from raw scores, correct the raw score bias against off-target changes and protect us from being misled by the unavoidable vagaries of mistargeting.

Figure 2, which shows two test curves spaced about 20 linear units apart, illustrates a situation in which the apparent advantage of a treatment effect on group A from A1 to A2 of 4 raw score points over a treatment effect on group B from B1 to B2 of only 2 raw score points is, in fact, reversed when these same raw scores are converted to equated linear measures. Now the advantage is with the six linear unit change of group B over the merely two linear unit change of group A.

This interpretation is confirmed when we examine the second dashed test curve centered at 20 linear units to the right of the solid test curve centered at zero. On this "harder" test, the targeted raw score increment for group B at 12 points is three times the targeted raw score increment for group A of only 4 points.

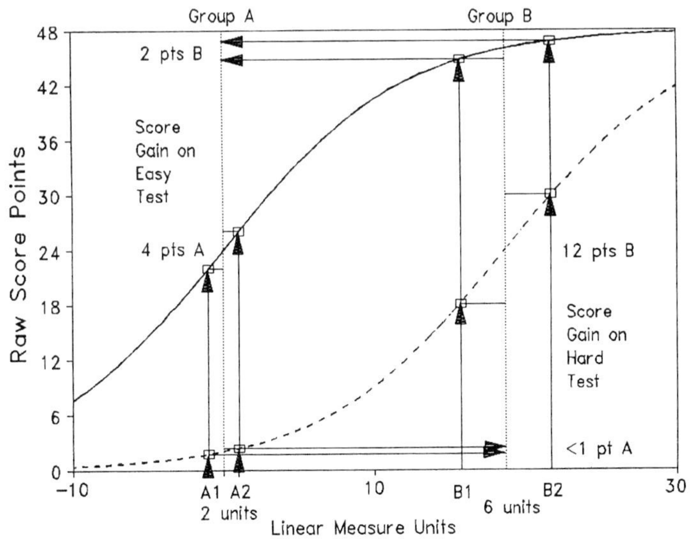

FIGURE 2. Measure changes can reverse raw score implications.

TABLE 1. Measure Increment Ratios for One More Right Answer at the Largest and Smallest Score Steps

Number of Steps*	Normal Test	Uniform Test
10	2.0	3.5
25	4.6	4.5
50	8.9	6.0
100	17.6	8.0

* For example, a seven-category rating scale supplies six steps per item; 13 such items produce 6 × 13 = 78 steps.
The ratio for a normal test of L items is: log{2(L-1)/L-2)}/log{(L+2)/L-2)}.
See Wright BD, Stone MH: Best Test Design: Rasch Measurement. Chicago, MESA Press, 1979.

This example shows that, when we rely on raw scores alone to judge the relative magnitude of outcome changes taking place at different distances from the center of the test curve, we can make conclusions so mistaken that they reverse our findings. We can conclude the opposite of what our data, when converted from ordinal raw scores to linear measures, make plain.

Table 1 documents the magnitude of raw score bias against extreme measures for a test of normally distributed item difficulties and a test of uniformly distributed item difficulties. The table uses ratios to compare the measure increment corresponding to one more rating step up at the next to largest extreme step with the measure increment corresponding to one more step up at the smallest central step.

Table 1 shows that even when items are spread in uniform increments of item difficulty, the raw score bias against measure increments at the extremes can easily be a factor of 5 or more. When items cluster in the middle of a test, the usual case, the bias can reach a factor of 10 or more. Should we research a comparison of outcome treatments, where the treatment effects are centered at different levels of functional independence, the less effective treatment could easily appear five times better than the more effective treatment simply because the treatment effects are targeted differently by the test we happen to use.

Raw score bias is not limited to dichotomous responses. Because of the effect of additional within-item steps, the bias is even more severe for partial credits, rating scales, and, of course, the Likert scale, the misuse of which pushed Thurstone's seminal 1920s work on how to transform raw scores into linear measures out of use.

These examples of raw score bias in favor of central scores and against extreme scores show that raw scores are target-biased and sample-dependent.[38–40] Any statistical method like linear regression, analysis of variance, generalizability, LISREL, or factor analysis that misuses nonlinear raw scores or Likert scales as though they were linear measures will have its output systematically distorted by this bias. Like the raw scores on which they are based, all results will be target-biased and sample-dependent and hence inferentially ambiguous. The obvious and easily practiced[16,37] law of measurement is: *Before applying linear statistical methods to concrete raw data, one must first use a measurement model to construct, from the observed raw data, abstract sample and test free linear measures.*

There are two additional advantages obtained by model-controlled linearization that are decisive for successful scientific research. Each measurement-model-estimated measure and calibration is accompanied by realistic estimates of *precision* and mean square residual-from-expectation evaluations of the extent to which their data patterns fit the measurement model, i.e., their statistical *validity*. When we plot

TABLE 2. Raw Scores Are Not Measures

Feature	Concrete Ordinal Raw Scores	Abstract Linear Measures
Additivity	Nonadditive Nonlinear *Bent*	Additive Linear *Straight*
Continuity	Discrete *Lumpy*	Continuous *Smooth*
Status	Incomplete *Raw*	Complete *Refined*
Control	Unsupervised Unvalidated *Wild*	Supervised Validated *Tamed*
Generality	Local Concrete Irreproducible *Test-bound*	General Abstract Reproducible *Test-free*

results and apply linear statistics to study relationships among measures, we not only have linear measures to work with but also know their precision and validity.

Table 2 summarizes the important differences between concrete ordinal raw scores and abstract interval linear measures.

• *Additivity* is the first difference. Without additivity one cannot use ordinary arithmetic to analyze results. One cannot apply the usual linear statistics of analysis of variance or regression without incurring the irresolvable ambiguities caused by raw score bias against off-target measures.

• *Continuity* is a second difference. Raw scores are forced to vary discontinuously in the integer steps, which correspond to one more and one less observation. Fractions are unobservable. Measures, on the other hand, being abstract representations of theoretical constructs, are continuous in our imagination and so too in our mathematical analyses. In practice, the values we can estimate for our measures are only as fine-grained as we can build measuring devices to approximate them. But that makes the discontinuity entirely a question of instrumentation engineering. Our ideas of our measures remain continuous.

• *Status* refers to the implacable reality that raw scores are limited to being nothing more than finite examples of what we are looking for and hence forever incomplete. Measures, on the other hand, in our stochastic conception of them, are complete ideas.

• *Control* refers to the opportunity when working with measures estimated from raw scores to compare the observation values expected from the measures by our measurement model with the observations actually obtained. This enables a continuous, on-line supervision of the empirical validity of our theoretical measures.

• *Generality* follows from interpreting raw data as an example of an enduring stochastic process that is closely governed by conjointly estimable measurement parameters. This is what enables us to take the inferential step from a finite concrete situation-bound experience to an infinitely reproducible abstract situation-liberated idea.

THE HISTORY OF FUNDAMENTAL MEASUREMENT

The ideas summarized in Table 2 draw us into the scientific history of fundamental measurement.

Concatenation

In 1920 English physicist Norman Campbell[5] deduced that the "fundamental" measurement (on which the success of physics was based) required, at least by analogy, the possibility of a physical concatenation, like joining the ends of sticks to concatenate length or piling bricks to concatenate weight.

Sufficiency

In 1920 English mathematician Ronald Fisher,[10] while developing his "likelihood" version of inverse probability to construct maximum likelihood estimation, discovered a statistic so "sufficient" that it exhausted all information concerning its modeled parameter from the data in hand. Statistics that exhaust all modeled information enable conditional formulations by which a value for each parameter can be estimated independently of all other parameters in the model. This necessity for the construction of fundamental measurement follows because the presence of a parameter in the model can be replaced by its sufficient statistic. Fisher's sufficiency enables independent parameter estimation for models that incorporate many different parameters.[1] This leads to a second law of measurement: *When a measurement model employs parameters for which there are no sufficient statistics, that model cannot construct useful measurement because it cannot estimate its parameters independently of one another.*

Divisibility

In 1924 French mathematician Paul Levy proved that the construction of an inferentially stable law required infinitely divisible parameters.[15] Levy's divisibility is logarithmically equivalent to the conjoint additivity[17] that we now recognize as the mathematical generalization of the concatenation Campbell required for fundamental measurement. Levy's conclusions were reinforced in 1932 when Russian mathematician A.N. Kolmogorov proved that independence of parameter estimates also required divisibility, this time in the form of an additive decomposition.[14]

Louis Thurstone's Contributions

Between 1925 and 1932 American electrical engineer Louis Thurstone published 24 articles and a book on the construction of psychological measures and developed mathematical methods that came close to satisfying every measurement requirement of which Thurstone was aware.

• **Unidimensionality**. The measurement of any object or entity describes only one attribute of the object measured. *This is a universal characteristic of all measurement.*[31]

• **Linearity**. The very idea of measurement implies a linear continuum of some sort such as length, price, volume, weight, age. When the idea of measurement is applied to scholastic achievement, for example, it is necessary to force the qualitative variations into a scholastic linear scale of some kind.[33]

• **Abstraction**. The linear continuum which is implied in all measurement is always an abstraction. . . . There is a popular fallacy that a unit of measurement is a thing—such as a piece of yardstick. This is not so. *A unit of measurement is always a process of some kind which can be repeated without modification in the different parts of the measurement continuum.*[31]

• **Sample free calibration**. *The scale must transcend the group measured.* One crucial test must be applied to our method of measuring attitudes before it can be accepted as valid. A measuring instrument must not be seriously affected in its measuring function by the object of measurement. . . . Within the range of objects . . . intended, its function must be independent of the object of measurement.[30]

• **Test free measurement**. It should be possible to omit several test questions at different levels of the scale *without affecting the individual score (measure). . . .* It should *not* be required to submit every subject to the whole range of the scale. The starting point and the terminal point . . . *should not directly affect the individual score (measure)*.[32]

Case V of Thurstone's Law of Comparative Judgement[29] is a fundamental measurement solution for the analysis of paired comparisons.

Louis Guttman's Contributions

In 1944 American sociologist Louis Guttman pointed out that the meaning of any raw score, including Likert scales, would remain ambiguous unless the score specified every response in the pattern on which it was based. Guttman wrote: "If a person endorses a more extreme statement, he should endorse *all* less extreme statements if the statements are to be considered a scale. . . . We shall call a set of items of common content a scale if [and only if] a person with a higher rank than another person is just as high or higher on *every* item than the other person."[13]

According to Guttman, only data that manifest this kind of perfect conjoint transitivity can produce unambiguous measures. Notice the similarity in motivation between Guttman's "scalability" and Ronald Fisher's "sufficiency." Both require that an unambiguous statistic must exhaust the information to which it is said to refer.

Georg Rasch's Contributions

In 1953 Danish mathematician Georg Rasch[20] found that the only way he could compare past performances on different tests of oral reading was to apply the exponential additivity of Poisson's 1837 distribution[27] to data produced by a new sample of students responding simultaneously to both tests. Rasch used Poisson because it was the only distribution he could think of that enabled the equation of the two tests to be entirely independent of the obviously arbitrary distribution of the reading abilities of the new sample.

As Rasch worked out his mathematical solution to what became an unexpectedly successful test equating, he discovered that the mathematics of the probability process, the measurement model, must be restricted to formulations that produced sufficient statistics. Only when his parameters had sufficient statistics could he use these statistics to remove the unwanted person parameters from his estimation equations and so obtain estimates of his test parameters that were independent of the values or distributions of whatever other parameters were at work in the measurement model.

Rasch's description of the conjoint transitivity he requires of the probabilities defined by his measurement model reveals that he has constructed a stochastic solution to the otherwise impossible problem of living up to Guttman's deterministic requirement for the existence of a useful rating scale. Rasch wrote: "A person having a greater ability than another should have the greater probability of solving *any* item of the type in question, and similarly, one item being more difficult than another one means that for *any* person the probability of solving the second item correctly is the greater one."[20]

In completing his measurement model, Rasch's "measuring function" specifies the multiplicative definition of fundamental measurement for dichotomous observations as:

$$f(P) \equiv b/d$$

Where P is the probability of a correct solution. f(P) is a function of P, still to be determined. b is a ratio measure of person ability. And d is a ratio calibration of item difficulty.

Rasch explains this model as an inverse probability.

> The model deals with the probability of a correct solution, which may be taken as the imagined outcome of an indefinitely long series of trials. . . . The formula says that in order that the concepts b and d could be at all considered meaningful, f(P), as derived in some way from P, should equal the ratio between b and d.[20]

And, after pointing out that a normal probit, even with its second parameter set to one, will be too "complicated" to serve as the measuring function f(P), asks: "Does there exist such a function, f(P), that f(P) = b/d is fulfilled?"[20]

Because "an additive system . . . is simpler than the original . . . multiplicative system." Rasch takes logarithms:

$$\log\{f(P)\} = \log b - \log d = B - D$$

which "for technical advantage" he expresses as the logit

$$L = \log\{P/(1 - P)\}$$

The question has now reached its final shape:[20] Does there exist a function g(L) of the variable L which forms an additive system in parameters for person B and parameters for items –D such that

$$g(L) = B - D$$

Asking "whether the measuring function for a test, if it exists at all, is uniquely determined, Rasch proves that

$$f(P) = C\{F_0(P)\}^A$$

"is a measuring function for any positive values of C and A, if $f_0(P)$ is so," which "contains all the possible measuring functions which can be constructed from $f_0(P)$." So that "By suitable choice of dimensions and units, i.e., of A and C for f(P), it is possible to make the b's and d's vary within any positive interval which may for some reason be deemed convenient."[20]

Because of "the validity of a separability theorem (sufficiency): It is possible to arrange the observational situation in such a way that from the responses of a number of persons to the set of items in question we may derive two sets of quantities, the distributions of which depend only on the item parameters, and only on the personal parameters, respectively. Furthermore the conditional distribution of the whole set of data for given values of the two sets of quantities does not depend on any of the parameters."[20]

> With respect to separability, the choice of this model has been lucky. Had we for instance assumed the "Normal-Ogive Model" with all $s_i = 1$, which numerically may be hard to distinguish from the logistic—then the separability theorem would have broken down. And the same would, in fact, happen for any other conformity model which is not equivalent in the sense of $f(P) = C\{f_0(P)\}^A$ to $f(P) = b/d$ . . . as regards separability. The possible distributions are limited to rather simple types but lead to rather far reaching generalizations of the Poisson process.[20]

By 1960 Rasch had proven that formulations in the compound Poisson family, such as Bernoulli's binomial, were both sufficient and, more surprising, necessary for the construction of stable measurement. Rasch had found that the "multiplicative Poisson" was the only mathematical solution to the second step in inference, the formulation of an objective, sample and test free measurement model.

The implications of Rasch's discovery have taken many years to reach practice.[18,34–36] Even today there are social scientists who do not understand or benefit from what Campbell, Levy, Kolmogorov, Fisher, and Rasch have proven.

Conjoint Additivity

The Americans working on mathematical foundations for measurement were unaware of Rasch's accomplishments. Their work came to a head with the proof by mathematical psychologists Duncan Luce and John Tukey that Campbell's concatenation was a physical realization of a general mathematical rule which, in its formulation, is "the" definition of fundamental measurement.[17] They called their formulation, which is necessary and sufficient for useful measurement, "conjoint additivity." They described conjoint additivity as follows:

> The essential character of . . . the fundamental measurement of extensive quantities is described by an axiomatization for the comparison of effects of arbitrary combinations of "quantities" of a *single specified kind*. . . . Measurement on a ratio scale follows from such axioms.
>
> The essential character of simultaneous conjoint measurement is described by an axiomatization for the comparison of effects of *pairs* formed from two specified kinds of "quantities". . . Measurement on interval scales which have a common unit follows from these axioms.
>
> A close relation exists between conjoint measurement and the establishment of response measures in a two-way table . . . for which the "effects of columns" and the "effects of rows" are additive. Indeed the discovery of such measures . . . may be viewed as the discovery, via conjoint measurement, of fundamental measures of the row and column variables.
>
> In spite of the practical advantages of such response measures, objections have been raised to their quest. . . . The axioms of simultaneous conjoint measurement overcome these objections. . . . Additivity is just as axiomatizable as concatenation . . . in terms of axioms that lead to . . . interval and ratio scales.
>
> In . . . the behavioral and biological sciences, where factors producing orderable effects and responses deserve more useful and more fundamental measurement, the moral seems clear: *when no natural concatenation operation exists, one should try to discover a way to measure factors and responses such the "effects" of different factors are additive.*

Although Luce and Tukey seem to have been unaware of Rasch's work, others noted:

"The Rasch model is a special case of additive conjoint measurement . . . a fit of the Rasch model implies that the cancellation axiom (i.e., conjoint transitivity) will be satisfied. . . . It then follows that items and persons are measured on an interval scale with a common unit."[4]

THE MEASUREMENT MODEL

Data come in the form of nominal response categories such as: *yes/no, present/absent, always/usually/sometimes/never, right/wrong, strongly agree/agree/*

disagree/strongly disagree. The labels for these categories suggest an ordering from less to more, more *yes*, more *presence*, more *occurrence*, more *rightness*, more *agreement*. We take for granted that this kind of labeling necessarily establishes a reliable hierarchy of ordinal response categories, an ordered rating scale. Whether empirical responses to such labels are, in fact, actually distinct or even in their expected order, however, remains to be discovered when the data are studied with an articulate measurement model.

It is not only the unavoidable ambiguity of what is counted or lack of knowledge as to the functioning distances between the ordered categories that mislead us. The response counts cannot form a linear scale. Not only are they restricted to occur as integers between none and all; not only are they systematically biased against off-target measures; but, because, at best, they are counts, their natural quantitative comparison will be as ratios rather than differences. Means and standard deviations calculated from these ranks are systematically misleading.

There are serious problems with initial raw data: ambiguity of entity, nonlinearity, and confusion of source (Is it the smart person or the easy item that produces the "right" answer?). In addition it is not these particular data that interest us. Our needs focus on what the data imply about future data, which, in the service of inference, are by definition "missing." We take the inverse probability step to inference by addressing each piece of observed data, x_{ni}, as a stochastic consequence of its modeled probability of occurring, P_{nix}.

We take the mathematical step to inference by connecting P_{nix} to a function that specifies how the measurement parameters in which we are interested might govern P_{nix}. Our parameters could be B_n, the location measure of person n on the continuum of reference; D_i, the location calibration of item i on the same continuum; and F_x, the threshold of the transition from category (x-1) to category (x).

The necessary and sufficient formulations then are:

$$P_{nix}/P_{nix-1} \equiv b_n/d_i f_x$$

and

$$\log(P_{nix}/P_{nix-1}) \equiv B_n - D_i - F_x$$

in which the symbol "≡" means "by definition" rather than merely "equals."

The first formulation shows how this model meets the Levy/Kolmogorov divisibility requirement. The second formulation shows how, in log odds form, this model meets the Campbell/Luce/Tukey conjoint additivity requirement. On the left is the replacement of x_{ni} by its Bernoulli/Bayes/Laplace stochastic proxy P_{nix}.

On the right of the second formulation we see the conjoint additivity that produces parameter estimates in the linear form to which our eyes, hands, and feet are so naturally accustomed.

When we want to see what we mean, we draw a picture because only seeing is believing. But the only pictures we see successfully are graphs of linear measures. Graphs of ratios mislead us; our eyes cannot "see" things that way. Needless to say, what we cannot see we cannot understand, let alone believe.

Indeed, Fechner showed that when we experience any kind of ratio—light, sound or pain—our nervous system "takes its logarithm" so that we can "*see* how it feels" on a linear scale.[9] Fechner was not the first to notice this neurologic phenomena. When tuned according to the Pythagorean scale, musical instruments sounded out of tune at each change of key. Pythagorean tuning was key-dependent. This inconvenience was resolved in the 17th century, 200 years before Fechner's work, by tuning instruments to notes that increased in frequency by equal ratios.

Equal ratio tuning produces an "equally tempered" scale of notes that sound equally spaced in any key and so are sufficiently "objective" to be "key-free," as it were. Bach's motive for writing "The Well-Tempered Clavier" was to demonstrate the value of this invention.

Inverse Probability in Practice

The use of inverse probability to implement inference redirects our attention away from seeking models to fit data toward finding data that fit the particular models by which we define measurement. Binomial transition odds like $P_{nijkx}/P_{nijkx-1}$ propel inferential meaning. Raw data are recorded in categories such as *right/wrong* and *agree/disagree*. We label these categories: X = 0, 1, 2, 3, 4, , , so that each X label counts a step up along the intended order of categories. For example, for *wrong*, X = 0; for *right*, X = 1. Or, for *strongly disagree*, X = 0; *disagree*, X = 1; *agree*, X = 2; *strongly agree*, X = 3.

We then connect X to the circumstances in which we are trying to measure by subscribing X, as in X_{nijk}, so that X_{nijk} can stand for a rating earned by performer n on item i from judge j for task k.

Then P_{nijkx} can be the inverse probability that performer n gets rated X on item i by judge j for task k.

The transition odds that the rating is X rather than X – 1 become $P_{nijkx}/P_{nijkx-1}$, as in:

	$P_{nijkx-1}$	P_{nijkx}	
X – 2	X – 1	X	X + 1

We then "explain" the logarithm of these transition odds as the consequence of a conjointly additive parameter composition like $B_n - D_i - C_j - A_k - F_x$ so that our measurement model becomes:

$$\log(P_{nijkx}/P_{nijkx-1}) \equiv B_n - D_i - C_j - A_k - F_x$$

This conjoint additivity provides inferential stability.

Three Essential Statistics and their Representation

To use measures wisely we need to know three things about every measure:

1. Its location on the linear measurement scale, *amount*.
2. Its range of reasonable values, *precision*.
3. Its empirical coherence, *validity*.

Finally, to "see" what our statistics mean, we need to:

4. Plot them into an informative *picture*.

To estimate the *amount* of the measure is, of course, our motivation for constructing it in the first place. But no measure, however carefully constructed, can be exact. There is always some error in the measure. We need to know how big this error is so that we can keep in mind the *precision* of the measure as we work with it.

There are two main sources of measurement error. The first is an intrinsic component of the stochasticity of our measurement model. The binomial basis for the inverse probability dictates an entirely expected level of measure error. The magnitude of this error component is governed, first by the number of replications, as in the number of observable steps or the number of rating forms completed, and, second, by the targeting of items on persons.

But that modeled and hence expected error is not all. We can only obtain data for measures in a real situation that is inevitably fraught with potentially interfering circumstances. We cannot know ahead of time how much these circumstances muddy the measures. Things are bound to be slightly different every time. Fortunately, the fit statistics of the measurement model give an excellent indication of how much unplanned for disturbance we actually encounter at each application.

Thus, a second error component, determined by the situation in which our raw data are obtained, which always decreases the actual precision of our measures, must be factored into the mathematically modeled precision to produce a realistic precision estimate.

Finally, the same fit statistics that help bring our measure precision into rapport with the actual situation in which the raw data were obtained also indicate the general validity of the measure. When the pattern of observed data comes close to the expected values predicted by the measurement model, we can see that the measure and its error are valid. But, when some of the observed values wander far from expectation, we cannot overlook the fact that something has interfered with the data collection and so made the measure less valid then we might have wished.

A useful feature of the comparisons between observed and expected raw responses is that the specificities of these discrepancies—which person, which item—often show what caused the interference and so suggest how we might control the intrusion of further interferences of this kind.

To illustrate, imagine that to evaluate my diet I weigh myself five times each morning and record the following readings from my bathroom scale:

On Monday I read:

	Pounds	*Mean*	*Error*	*Range*
	180			
MON	179	180	± 1	178–182
	178			
	181		Results that are	
	182		*valid* and *precise*	

The five readings cluster nicely. It is obvious that 180 is a rather precise estimate of my Monday weight—to the nearest pound.

On Tuesday, however, the weights are different:

	Pounds	*Mean*	*Error*	*Range*
	180			
TUES	175	180	± 5	*170–190*
	170			
	185		Results that are still	
	190		*valid* and somewhat *imprecise!*	

The way I used my scale on Tuesday was obviously not as accurate as on Monday. Am I jumping on the scale too roughly? My best Tuesday estimate of my weight is still 180, but now only to the nearest 5 pounds, perhaps too crude to detect any success from my diet.

So, on Wednesday I am careful how I step on the scale, but something else goes wrong:

	Pounds	*Mean*	*Error*	*Range*
	177			
WED	174	180	*? ? ?*	*173–200*
	200			
	176		These results must	
	173		be *invalid!*	

One of my five weighings does not make sense. How could I suddenly weigh 20 pounds more? Was that the moment my wife, trying to see how much I weighed, leaned on my shoulder as I stood on the scale? One thing for sure, that reading of 200 is out of line with the other four readings and has to be reconsidered.

Now, look at how nice and sensible my results become when I omit that wild 200:

	Pounds	*Mean*	*Error*	*Range*
	177			
WED	174	175	± 1	173–177
	176			
	173		Once again, both *valid* and *precise*	

And, glory be, I'm 5 pounds lighter! My diet is working!

We discovered the measurement hazards in this story by reading the numbers carefully. But reading numbers takes concentration; few do it well. I'll bet that, had I not dramatized that errant "200," you might have missed it and come to the wrong conclusion about the success of my diet. To avoid the easy mistake of misreading tables of numbers, it is always a good idea to make a picture of the numbers in some kind of plot. Plots of numbers are always better than tables.

Let's see what my weighings look like when I plot them. Figure 3 tells the story at a glance—no need to read anything carefully. The increase of uncertainty from Monday to Tuesday is obvious and the irregularity of that 200 on Wednesday is glaring. Neither can be missed. You can also see directly that once the 200 is excluded from Wednesday's readings, Wednesday's precision is as good as Monday's and that I have definitely lost some weight.

Why did I weigh myself five times each morning? By now you should be able to answer that question easily. What if I had weighed myself only once and that one reading turned out to be the 200? How misled I would have been. Ask yourself the same question in a more dramatic context. How many tosses of my "lucky quarter"

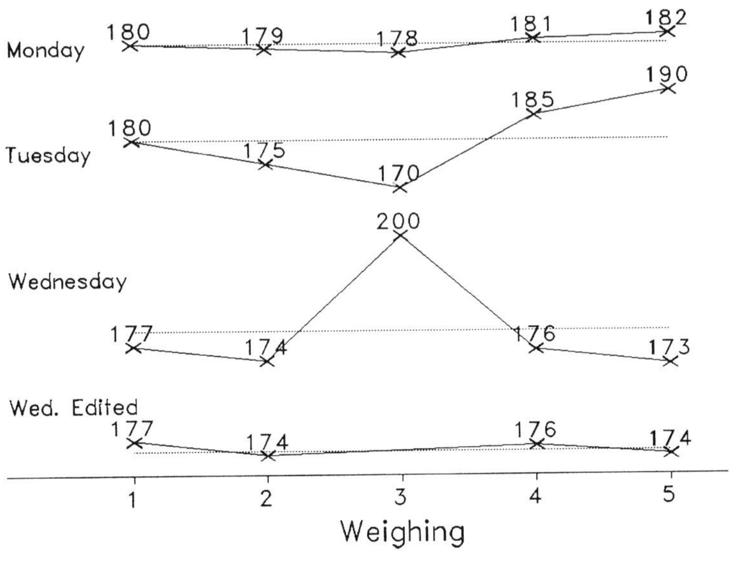

FIGURE 3. Three days on Ben's bathroom scale.

would you demand to check for fairness before you bet your life on it? Would once or twice be enough? Not likely!

What does that mean about scores and measures? One observation, one score from one item is never enough! Neither is one second opinion enough! To make a wise or even sensible decision, we must obtain several independent replications of the relevant measures before we act.

To summarize:

• We need *measures* not scores, or change is without evidence.

• We need to know the *precision* of the measures, or their implications remain obscure.

• We need to verify the *validity* of the measurement process by obtaining several independent replications, or meaning is uncertain.

• No matter how smart we are, we need more than one observation, more than one opinion. We need *replications*.

• Finally, a plot is worth a thousand numbers. A good *picture* may be the only way to "see" what a set of numbers means.

A FUNDAMENTAL MEASURE FOR APPLIED SELF-CARE

To perform this kind of analysis, category ratings are recorded on disk and analyzed with computer programs, such as BIGSTEPS or *FACETS*.[16,37] This kind of analysis gives tables, maps, keys, and files of conjoint linear measures.

The following example of Rasch BIGSTEPS analysis comes from 3128 administrations of the eight-item PECS Applied Self-Care LifeScale. This scale evaluates eight aspects of self-care: a bowel program, urinary program, skin care program, health cognizance, health activity, health education, safety awareness, and medication knowledge. A nurse is asked to rate the patient's competence on each of the eight items according to a seven-category rating scale intended to bring out gradients of competence for each item (Table 3). For example, in the bowel program, effectiveness concerns regulation of bowel elimination and prevention of complications includes regulation of food and fluids, high-fiber diet, medications for stimulation or prevention of diarrhea, digital stimulation, and colostomy care.

The data matrix has 3128 rows, a row for each patient n, and 8 columns, a column for each item i. The cell entry x_{ni} is an ordinal rating from 1 to 7 of patient n on item i. BIGSTEPS analyzes this matrix of 25,024 raw data points to produce the best possible (1) 8-item calibrations to define the PECS applied self-care construct; (2) for each item, 6 rating step calibrations to its step structure; and (3) 3,128 measures of the extent of each patient's self-care.

TABLE 3. Rating Scale of PECS Applied Self-Care LifeScale

Rating		Category Definition
1	Ineffective	Less than 25% effective
2	Dependent	25%–49% effective
3	Dependent	50%–74% effective
4	Dependent	75%–100% effective
5	Independent	50%–74% effective
6	Independent	75%–100% effective
7	Normal	Self maintenance

TABLE 4. Summary of the BIGSTEPS Analysis of the PECS LifeScales: Applied Self-Care

Entered: 3128 Patients   Analyzed: 2145 Patients   8 Items   56 Categories

Summary of 2145 Measured (Non-extreme) Patients

	Raw Score	Count	Measure	Model Error	Infit MNSQ	Outfit MNSQ	
Mean	26.2	7.5	41.56	4.94	.88	.89	
S.D.	11.0	.9	22.09	1.35	1.06	1.10	

Model RMSE	5.12	Adj. SD	21.49	Separation	4.19	Reliability	.95
Real RMSE	5.80	Adj. SD	21.32	Separation	3.68	Reliability	.93
S.E. of Person Mean		.48					

Maximum Extreme Score: 5 Patients   Minimum Extreme Score: 94 Patients
Lacking Responses: 884 Patients   Valid Responses: 94.3%

Summary of 8 Measured (Non-extreme) Items

	Raw Score	Count	Measure	Model Error	Infit MNSQ	Outfit MNSQ	
Mean	7034.1	2023.1	50.01	.28	.83	.88	
S.D.	829.2	148.5	4.83	.02	.23	.24	

Model RMSE	.29	Adj. SD	4.82	Separation	16.91	Reliability	1.00
Real RMSE	.29	Adj. SD	4.82	Separation	16.64	Reliability	1.00
S.E. of Person Mean		1.82					

Output from BIGSTEPS (Wright, B.D., Linacre, J.M. 1997)

The analysis not only extracts the best possible linear measurement framework but also reduces the complexity of the data from 25,024 raw ordinal data points to a mere 8 item calibrations + 48 item step calibrations + 3,128 person measures, all 3,184 of which estimates are expressed in linear metrics on a common scale that measures a single dimension of "self-care" (Table 4).

What follows are excerpts from a BIGSTEPS analysis of these data. Readers are not expected to master every detail shown in these excerpts. Instead, sit back and notice, to whatever extent is comfortable for you, the various ways this kind of analysis can bring inevitably complicated data into a few well-organized tables and pictures.

Table 4 summarizes the results of this 87% reduction of the raw ordinal data and describes the summary characteristics of its reconstruction into a unidimensional measurement framework. Table 4 contains two important points:

1. 2145 patients are measured at nonextreme scores, and among these ratings are completion is 94.3%.
2. The reliability of this 8-item scale to separate the self-care measures of these 2145 patients is a high 0.93.

To see the meaning of the BIGSTEPS definition of the PECS self-care construct, we plot the item calibrations and patient measures together on the MAP in Figure 4. The left column benchmarks the linear units of the measurement framework scale for this analysis to run from –20 to 120. The MAP is focused on the region from 0 to 90.

The second column shows the frequency distribution of the 2096 patients who measure between 0 and 90. The symbols M, S, and Q mark the mean patient measure at M, plus and minus one standard deviation at each S and plus and minus two standard deviations at each Q. Finally, on the right, six of the eight items defining this

```
MEASURE    PATIENTS          RATING.APPLIED SELF-CARE
--------------------------------------------------------------
  90                .  +             6.KNOWS MEDICATIONS
                    .  |
                   .# Q|             6.HEALTH ACTIVITY
                    .  |             6.SAFETY AWARENESS
  80              .##  +             6.SKIN CARE PROGRAM
                 .###  |             6.BOWEL PROGRAM
                  .##  |             6.URINARY PROGRAM
               .#####  |
  70             .###  +
               .#####  |
            #########  |
            ######### S|
  60        .########  +         4.KNOWS MEDICATIONS
          .##########  |
                .####  |         4.HEALTH ACTIVITY
          .##########  |         4.SAFETY AWARENESS
  50           .#####  +         4.SKIN CARE PROGRAM
             .#######  |         4.BOWEL PROGRAM
                #####  |         4.URINARY PROGRAM
             ######## M|
  40   .############   +     3.KNOWS MEDICATIONS
         .###########  |
           .#########  |     3.HEALTH ACTIVITY
              .######  |     3.SAFETY AWARENESS
  30          .######  +     3.SKIN CARE PROGRAM
             .#######  |     3.BOWEL PROGRAM
             .#######  |     3.URINARY PROGRAM
              .######  |
  20           .##### S+
              .######  |
               .#####  |
                .####  | 1.KNOWS MEDICATIONS
  10            .####  +
                   .#  | 1.HEALTH ACTIVITY
                    .  | 1.SAFETY AWARENESS
                  .##  | 1.SKIN CARE PROGRAM
   0               .#  + 1.BOWEL PROGRAM
                 .### Q| 1.URINARY PROGRAM
--------------------------------------------------------------
```

OUTPUT FROM BIGSTEPS (WRIGHT, B.D. & LINACRE, J.M. 1997)

FIGURE 4. A MAP of PECS LifeScales: applied self-care.

self-care construct are shown in their calibration order four times, once at each of the rating levels 1 at "Ineffective," 3 and 4 at "Dependent," and 6 at "Independent."

This was done to show how this definition of self-care moves up from ratings of *ineffectiveness* in the 0 to 10 measure region, through two successive levels of *dependence* in the 25 to 60 measure region, to ratings of *independence* in the 75 to 90 measure region.

Figure 4 shows only six of the eight items because *medications* and *education* calibrate on top of each other at the same high level as do *skin care* and *cognizance* a bit lower down.

The mapped hierarchy of the six items begins with the *urinary* and *bowel* programs, which are the easiest to rate well on, and moves up through *skin care* (and *cognizance*), *safety* and *activity* to reach *medications* (and *education*), which are the hardest self-care programs to rate well on.

The practical application of this empirical hierarchy is that self-care education has the best chance of success when it begins at the easy end with *urinary* and *bowel* programs and only reaches up to the more challenging *activity* and *medications* programs after the easier programs are well established.

Table 5 lists the item calibrations from which the right side of Figure 4 was mapped. This table shows all eight items in their difficulty order and lists their

TABLE 5. Calibrations for the Eight Items Defining PECS LifeScales: Applied Self-Care

Items Statistics: Measure Order								
Entry Num	Raw Score	Count	Measure	Error	INFIT MNSQ	OUTFIT MNSQ	PTBIS	Hardest Item
8	5964	1866	57.4	.3	.96	.97	.82	Knows medications
6	5828	1832	57.1	.3	.66	.68	.89	Health education
5	6294	1800	52.1	.3	.72	.74	.87	Health activity
7	7458	2137	48.9	.3	.71	.78	.86	Safety awareness
4	7413	2135	48.2	.3	.47	.49	.91	Health cognizance
3	7290	2139	48.1	.3	1.22	1.29	.77	Skin care program
1	7858	2141	44.6	.3	.82	.92	.83	Bowel program
2	8168	2135	43.7	.3	1.09	1.16	.80	Urinary program
Mean	7034.	2023.	50.0	.3	.83	.88		Easiest item
S.D.	829.	148.	4.8	.0	.23	.24		

Input: 3128 patients, 8 items
Analyzed: 2145 patients, 8 items, 56 categories
Output from BIGSTEPS (Wright, B.D. & Linacre, J.M., 1997)

calibrations measures, estimation errors, and fit statistics by which the validity of these calibrations can be judged. The fit statistics, which have expected values of 1.00, show that the only item afflicted with calibration uncertainty is the *skin care* program item with mean square residual ratios of 1.22 and 1.29.

These fit statistics suggest that skin care may sometimes interact idiosyncratically with characteristics such as age, sex or impairment. Further examination of other BIGSTEPS output can be used to identify the particular patients who manifest the effects of such an interaction and hence bring out the individual diagnostics most helpful to these particular patients.

The analysis of the extent to which any particular set of data cooperates with a measurement model to define a desired variable and estimate useful measures along that variable is decisive in the construction of good measures. This topic is extensively and articulately explained in the published work of Richard Smith.[22–26]

Figure 5 illustrates the way BIGSTEPS analyzes how this set of categories are used to obtain patient ratings on each item. The item chosen here is the easiest, the *bowel* program. The plot in the top half of Figure 5 shows how the probabilities of category use from 1 up to 7 move to the right across the variable from low measures at –25 to high measures at +115. Each rating category in sequence has a modal region of greatest probability except for categories 5 and 6, which are underused on this item. This observation about the usage of categories 5 and 6 could lead us to question their distinction and, perhaps, to consider combining them into one category of "independence."

Below the plot is the frequency distribution of the 8567 patient ratings used for this analysis. At the bottom are observed counts, step difficulty calibrations, and measures expected at each rating level from 1 to 7. In the column Observed Count, the uses of categories 5 and 6, at counts of 860 and 727, fall far below the uses of category 4, at a count of 2503. That is why the curves for those two categories do not surface at the top of Figure 5.

Figure 6 gives the same information for the hardest item, *education*. The measure scale under the plot has moved up 12 units, and the step difficulties and expected

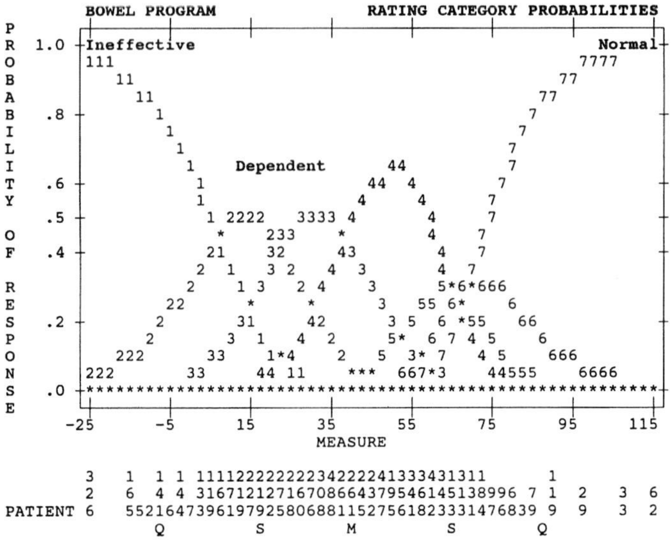

BOWEL PROGRAM **RATING STEP CALIBRATIONS**

CATEGORY LABEL	STEP VALUE	OBSERVED COUNT	STEP MEASURE	STEP ERROR	EXPECTED SCORE MEASURES STEP-.5	AT STEP	STEP+.5
Ineffective	1	618	NONE			(-6)	13
2	2	1049	7	.6	13	13	22
Dependent	3	1794	21	.4	22	30	40
4	4	2503	38	.3	40	50	58
Independent	5	860	66	.4	58	63	67
6	6	727	66	.4	67	72	78
Normal	7	1010	70	.5	78	(84)	
			mode			mean	

Output from BIGSTEPS (Wright, B.D. & Linacre, J.M. 1997)

FIGURE 5. Rating category step structure PECS LifeScales: applied self-care construct.

measures have increased. In the category curves for this item, every category has some importance. We would not be tempted to combine any of these categories.

Maps and summaries of item and category performance are essential to the analysis of the measurement quality of the test. But the ultimate aim is the measurement and diagnosis of each patient. This concern brings us to the diagnostic KEY forms illustrated in Figures 7 and 8.

After the construct MAP of Figure 4, KEY forms are the second most useful outcome of a BIGSTEPS analysis. Figure 7 shows two patients who received the same rating scores of 36 raw score points but who differ decisively in the best estimates of their self-care measures and who also differ in the diagnostic implications of their particular self-care ratings.

The typical patient at the top of Figure 7 measures at 60 self-care units, which is at the 70th percentile among a normative group of 8561 patients. This patient is verging on self-care independence except for the need for some additional help with the hardest programs, medication and education.

However, the atypical patient at the bottom of Figure 7, with the same raw score, appears differently when recorded on the patient's own KEY form. When the abysmal ineffectiveness in the medication and education programs is set aside, the

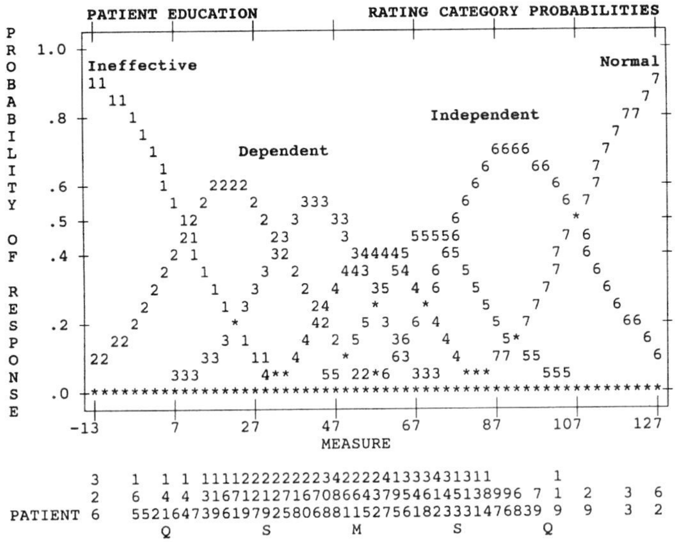

PATIENT EDUCATION — RATING STEP CALIBRATIONS

CATEGORY LABEL	STEP VALUE	OBSERVED COUNT	STEP MEASURE	STEP ERROR	EXPECTED SCORE MEASURES STEP-.5	AT STEP	STEP+.5
Ineffective	1	849	NONE			(-1)	18
2	2	1727	11	.5	18	22	33
Dependent	3	2018	33	.4	33	42	50
4	4	1403	50	.4	50	57	64
Independent	5	1233	63	.4	64	70	79
6	6	799	86	.5	79	92	108
Normal	7	92	107	1.2	108	(118)	
			mode			mean	

Output from BIGSTEPS (Wright, B.D. & Linacre, J.M. 1997)

FIGURE 6. Rating category step structure PECS LifeScales: applied self-care construct.

patient measures up at 73 units and the 85th percentile. The patient is well into independence on everything except education and medication. But, in those two aspects of self-care, the patient is dramatically deficient. The self-care education must concentrate on the earliest levels of these two areas.

Figure 8 shows a KEY form for another construct, *cognition and communication*. The patient is also atypical—this time in a way that implies a particular diagnosis. The deficiencies for this patient, in *short-term memory*, *attention/concentration*, and *orientation* suggest the possibility of Alzheimer's disease.

When a firm well-labeled frame of reference is constructed, we can then become aware of and attend to idiosyncratic aspects of the patient's status. The two patients represented in Figure 7 are not treated the same because they happen to have the same raw scores of 36. On the contrary, when a frame of reference is established, we can ask about more than the score. When the pattern of ratings contains values that, because of the structure of our measurement frame of reference, are unexpected, we can identify and respond to the details of the patient's personal needs.

In summary:

1. **Ratings are chancy**, but they are all we can observe. They may contain good information, but it is always in a "fuzzy" state.

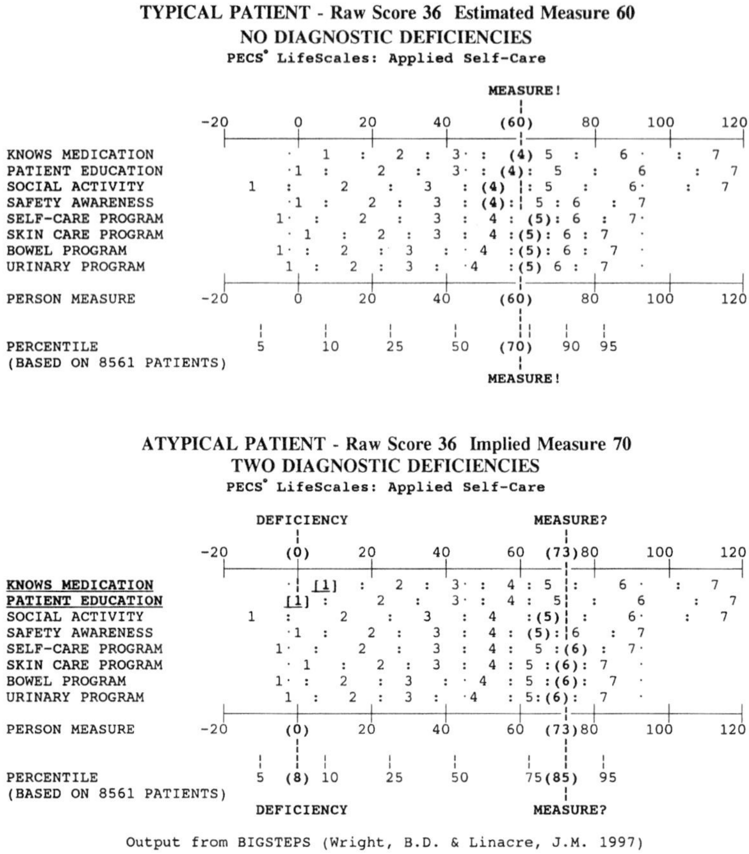

FIGURE 7. KEY forms for a typical and an atypical patient.

2. **Raw scores are not measures**. Raw scores are biased against off-target performance, are sample-dependent, inferentially unstable, and nonlinear.

3. **Inverse probability** explained by **conjointly additive parameters** enables the construction of clear measures from fuzzy raw scores.

4. These measures, in turn, enable the development of **MAPs**, which define the variable in a one-page, easily understood graphical report on the construct that the analysis has realized as a measurable variable.

5. The measures also enable the development of individual **KEYs**, which apply the variable sensitively and individually to each person to bring out the patient's personal information in an easily understood one-page graphical report.

CONCLUSION

A weight of seven was a tenet of faith among seventh century Muslims. Muslim leaders were censured for using less "righteous" standards.[21] Caliph of the Muslim world, 'Umar b. 'Abd al-'Aziz, instructs his governors that: "The people have been struck with trial, hardship, oppressive governments and wicked practices set upon them by evil tax collectors. The more righteous law is justice and

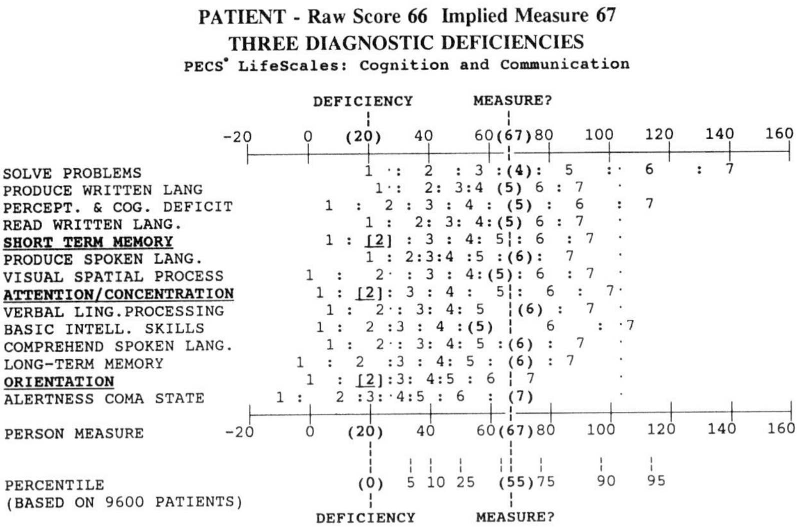

Output from BIGSTEPS (Wright, B.D. & Linacre, J.M. 1997)

FIGURE 8. Diagnostic KEY form for an Alzheimer patient.

good conduct. . . . I order you to take in taxes only the weight of seven." (Damascus, 723)

The Magna Carta of John, King of England, requires: "There shall be one measure of wine throughout Our kingdom, and one of ale, and one measure of corn, to wit, the London quarter, and one breadth of cloth, . . . , to wit, two ells within the selvages. As with measures so shall it be with weights." (Runnymede, 1215)

Thus, commerce and politics were the first source of stable units for length, area, volume, and weight. The steam engine added temperature and pressure. The subsequent successes of science stand on these commercial and engineering achievements. When we recall the long-standing political and moral history of units of taxation and trade we realize that when units are unequal, when they vary from time to time and place to place, it is not only unfair but immoral. So too with the misuse of necessarily unequal and, so, unfair raw score units when they are analyzed as though they were fair measures.

The main purpose of measurement is inference. We measure to inform and specify our plans for what to do next. If the measures are unreliable and the units vary in unknown ways, our plans must go astray. This point might seem small. Indeed, it has been belittled by many, presumably knowledgeable, social scientists as not worth worrying about. But, far from being a small point, it is a decisive one! We will not build a useful, let alone moral, social science until we stop deluding ourselves by analyzing raw scores as though they were measures.

INFERENCE

The concrete measures that help make life better are so familiar that we seldom think about "how" or "why" they work. Although the mathematics of measurement did not initiate its practice, it is the mathematics of measurement that provide the ultimate foundation for practice and the final logic by which useful measurement evolves and thrives. A mathematical history of measurement, however, takes us behind concrete practice to the theoretical requirements that make the practical success of measurement possible. There we discover that:

1. Measures are *inferences*,
2. Obtained by *stochastic approximations*,
3. Of *one-dimensional* quantities,
4. Counted in *abstract* units, of sizes that are
5. Intended to be *undisturbed* by extraneous factors.

To meet these requirements mathematically: *Measurement must be an inference of values for infinitely divisible parameters which define the transition odds between observable increments of a theoretical variable.*

Table 6 summarizes an anatomy of inference according to four obstacles that stand between raw data and the stable inference of measures they might imply.

Uncertainty is the motivation for inference. The future is uncertain by definition. We have only the past by which to foresee. Our solution is to capture uncertainty in a skein of imaginary probability distributions which regularize the irregularities that disrupt connections between what seems certain now but is certainly uncertain later. We call this step "inverse probability."

Distortion interferes with the transition from observation to conceptualization. Our ability to figure things out comes from our faculty to visualize. Our power of visualization evolved from the survival value of body navigation through the two-dimensional space in which we live. Our antidote to distortion is to represent our observations of experience in the linear form that makes them look like the space in front of us. To "see" what experience "means," we "map" it.

Confusion is caused by interdependencies. As we look for tomorrow's probabilities in yesterday's lessons, confusing interactions intrude. Our resolution of confusion is to simplify the complexity we experience into a few shrewdly crafted "dimensions." The authority of these dimensions is their utility. Final "truths" are unknowable. But, when our inventions work, we find them "useful." And when they continue to work, we come to believe in them and call them "real" and "true."

TABLE 6. An Anatomy of Inference

Obstacles	Solutions	Inventors
Uncertainty	**Probability**	Bernoulli 1713
have ⇨ want	binomial odds	Bayes 1764
now ⇨ later	regular irregularity	Laplace 1774
statistic ⇨ parameter	misfit detection	Poisson 1837
Distortion	**Additivity**	Fechner 1860
non-linearity	linearity	Helmholtz 1887
unequal intervals	concatenation	N. Campbell 1920
incommensurability	conjoint additivity	Luce/Tukey 1964
Confusion	**Separability**	Rasch 1958
interdependence	sufficiency	R.A. Fisher 1920
interaction	invariance	Thurstone 1925
confounding	conjoint order	Guttman 1944
Ambiguity	**Divisibility**	Levy 1924
of entity, interval	independence	Kolmogorov 1932
and aggregation	stability	Bookstein 1992

For information on Bernoulli, Bayes, Laplace, Poisson, and Helmholtz see Stigler SM: The History of Statistics. Cambridge, Harvard University Press, 1986.

The method we use to control confusion is to enforce unidimensionality. We define and measure one invented dimension at a time. The necessary mathematics is parameter separability. Models that introduce putative "causes" as separately estimable parameters are our laws of quantification. These models define measurement, determine what is measurable, decide which data are useful, and expose data that are not.

Ambiguity, a fourth obstacle to inference, occurs because we can never determine exactly which particular definitions of existential entities are the "right" ones. As a result, the only measurement models that can work are models that are indifferent to levels of composition. Bookstein[3] shows that to accomplish this the models must embody parameter divisibility or additivity as in:

$$H(xy) = H(x)H(y) \text{ and } G(x + y) = G(x) + G(y)$$

Fortunately the mathematical solutions to *ambiguity*, *confusion*, and *distortion* are identical. The parameters that govern the probabilities of the data must appear in either a divisible or additive form.

Inverse Probability

A critical turning point in the mathematical history of measurement is the application of Jacob Bernoulli's 1713 binomial distribution as an inverse probability for interpreting the implications of observed events.[27] The data are least of what we seek. Our interests go beyond to what these data imply about other data still unmet but important to foresee. When we read our weight as 180 pounds, we take that number, not as a one-time, local description of a particular stepping on the scale, but as our weight for now, just before now, and, inferentially, for awhile to come.

The first problem of inference is how to infer values for these other data, which, by the meaning of "inference," are currently "missing." Since the purpose of inference is to estimate what future data might be like before they occur, methods that require complete data cannot be methods of inference. This realization engenders a third law of measurement: *Any statistical method nominated to serve inference which requires complete data, by this requirement, disqualifies itself as an inferential method.*

But, if what we want to know is "missing," how can we use the data in hand to make useful inferences about the "missing" data they might imply? Inverse probability reconceives our raw observations as a probable consequence of a relevant stochastic process with a useful formulation. The apparent determinism of formulae like F = MA depends on the prior construction of relatively precise measures of F and A. The first step from raw observation to inference is to identify the stochastic process by which an inverse probability can be defined. Bernoulli's binomial distribution is the simplest and most widely used process. Mathematical analysis proves that the compound Poisson is the parent of all such measuring distributions.

Conjoint Additivity

The second step to inference is to discover what mathematical models can determine the stochastic process in a way that enables a stable, ambiguity resilient estimation of the model's parameters from the data in hand. At first glance, this step looks secure. Its 20th century history has followed so many paths, traveled by so many mathematicians and physicists that one might suppose there were no clear second step but only a jumble of unconnected possibilities along with their seemingly separate mathematical resolutions. Fortunately, reflection on the motivations for these paths and examination of their mathematics leads to a reassuring simplification. Although each path was motivated by a particular concern as to what inference must overcome to succeed, all solutions end up with the same simple, easy-to-understand, easy-to-use formulation. The mathematical function that governs the inferential stochastic process must specify parameters which are either *infinitely divisible* or *conjointly additive*, i.e., *separable*. That's all there is to it.

Some fundamental laws of measurement emerge as we explore the definition and necessities of inference: *Any statistical method nominated to serve inference which turns out to require complete data, by this very requirement, disqualifies itself as an inferential method.*

When a model employs parameters for which there are no sufficient statistics, that model cannot construct useful measurement because it cannot estimate its parameters independently.

Before applying linear statistical methods to raw data, one must first use a measurement model to construct, from the observed raw data, coherent sample and test free linear measures.

Practical solutions to Thurstones' five requirements include the following:

1. Measures must be linear, so that arithmetic can be done with them.
2. Item calibrations must not depend on whose responses are used to estimate them; they must be sample free.
3. Person measures must not depend on which items they happened to take; they must be test free.
4. Missing data must not matter.
5. The method must be easy to apply.

These requirements were latent in Campbell's 1920 analysis of concatenation,[5] Fisher's 1920 invention of sufficiency,[10] and the functional divisibility of Levy[15] and Kolmogorov.[14] Stable inference theory was realized practically by Rasch's 1953 application of the additive Poisson model to the equation of alternative tests of oral reading.[19]

Rasch's original model has since been extended to address every imaginable kind of raw observation: dichotomies, rating scales, partial credits, binomial and Poisson counts[18] in every reasonable observational situation, i.e., ratings faceted to persons, items, judges, and tasks. Today versatile computer programs make thorough applications of Rasch's "measuring functions" so easy, immediate, and accessible to every student of outcome measurement that there is no excuse for stopping analysis at a misconstruction of raw scores.

Despite hesitation by some to use a fundamental measurement model to transform raw scores into measures so that subsequent statistical analysis can become fruitful, there have been many successful applications,[11] and convenient software to accomplish these applications is readily available.[16,37]

Today, it is easy for any reasonably knowledgeable scientist to use these programs to traverse the decisive step from their unavoidably ambiguous concrete raw observations to well-defined abstract linear measures with realistic precision and validity estimates. There is no methodologic reason why outcome measurement cannot become as stable, as reproducible, and hence as useful as physics.

The mathematical knowledge needed to construct objective, fundamental measures from raw scores has been with us for more than 40 years. Easy-to-use computer programs that do the number work have been available for 30 years. What could possibly justify continuing to misuse raw scores as though they were measures when we know that they are not?

REFERENCES

1. Andersen EB: Sufficient statistics and latent trait models. Psychometrika 42:69–81, 1977.
2. Bookstein A: Informetric distributions. III. Ambiguity and randomness. J Am Soc Inform Sci 48:2–10, 1996.
3. Bookstein A: Informetric distributions. Parts I and II. J Am Soc Inform Sci 41:368–388, 1992.
4. Brogden HE: The Rasch model, the law of comparative judgement and additive conjoint measurement. Psychometrika 42:631–634, 1977.
5. Campbell NR: Physics: The Elements. London, Cambridge University Press, 1920.
6. Engelhard G: Historical views of the concept of invariance in measurement theory. In Wilson M (ed): Objective Measurement: Theory into Practice. Norwood, NJ, Ablex, 1994, pp 73–99.
7. Engelhard G: Thorndike, Thurstone and Rasch: A comparison of their approaches to item-invariant measurement. J Res Dev Educ 24:45–60, 1991.
8. Engelhard G: Thorndike, Thurstone and Rasch: A comparison of their methods of scaling psychological tests. Appl Psychol Measure 8:21–38, 1984.
9. Fechner GT: Elemente der Psychophysik. Leipzig, Breitkopf & Hartel, 1860 [Translation: Adler HE: Elements of Psychophysics. New York, Holt, Rinehart & Winston, 1966].
10. Fisher RA: A mathematical examination of the methods of determining the accuracy of an observation by the mean error and by the mean square error. Monthly Notices of the Royal Astronomical Society 53:758–770, 1920.
11. Fisher WP, Wright BD: Applications of probabilistic conjoint measurement. Special Issue. Int J Educ Res 21:557–664, 1994.
12. Guttman L: A basis for scaling quantitative data. Am Sociol Rev 9:139–150, 1944.
13. Guttman L: The basis for scalogram analysis. In Stouffer SA, et al (eds): Measurement and Prediction. Vol 4. Princeton, NJ, Princeton University Press, 1950, pp 60–90.
14. Kolmogorov AN: Foundations of the Theory of Probability. New York, Chelsea Publishing, 1950.
15. Levy P: Theorie de l'addition des variables aleatoires. Paris, 1937.
16. Linacre JM, Wright BD: FACETS: Many-Faceted Rasch Analysis. Chicago, MESA Press, 1997.
17. Luce RD, Tukey JW: Simultaneous conjoint measurement. J Math Psychol 1:1–27, 1964.
18. Masters GN, Wright BD: The essential process in a family of measurement models. Psychometrika 49:529–544, 1984.
19. Perline R, Wright BD, Wainer H: The Rasch model as additive conjoint measurement. Appl Psychol Measure 3:237–255, 1979.
20. Rasch G: Probabilistic Models for Some Intelligence and Attainment Tests. Chicago, MESA Press, 1993 [originally published in 1960 by the Danish Institute of Educational Research].
21. Sears SD: A Monetary History of Iraq and Iran [PhD dissertation]. Chicago, University of Chicago, 1997.
22. Smith RM: A comparison of the power of Rasch total and between item fit statistics to detect measurement disturbances. Educ Psychol Measure 54:42–55, 1994.
23. Smith RM: Person fit in the Rasch model. Educ Psychol Measure 46:359–372, 1986.
24. Smith RM: The distributional properties of Rasch item fit statistics. Educ Psychol Measure 51:541–565, 1991.
25. Smith RM: The distributional properties of Rasch standardized residuals. Educ Psychol Measure 48:657–667, 1988.
26. Smith RM: Validation of individual test response patterns. In International Encyclopedia of Education. Oxford, Pergamon Press, 1985, pp 5410–5413.
27. Stigler SM: The History of Statistics. Cambridge, Harvard University Press, 1986.
28. Thorndike EL: An Introduction to the Theory of Mental and Social Measurements. New York, Teacher's College, Columbia University, 1904.
29. Thurstone LL: A law of comparative judgement. Psychol Rev 34:273–286, 1927.
30. Thurstone LL: Attitudes can be measured. Am J Sociol 23:529–554, 1928.
31. Thurstone LL: Measurement of social attitudes. J Abnorm Soc Psychol 26:249–269, 1931.
32. Thurstone LL: The scoring of individual performance. J Educ Psychol 17:446–457, 1926.
33. Thurstone LL, Chave EJ: The Measurement of Attitude. Chicago, University of Chicago Press, 1929.
34. Wright BD: Despair and hope for educational measurement. Contemp Educ Rev 1:281–288, 1984.
35. Wright BD: Sample-free test calibration and person measurement. In Proceedings, 1967 Invitational Conference on Testing. Princeton, Educational Testing Service, 1968, pp 85–101.
36. Wright BD: Solving measurement problems with the Rasch model. J Educ Measure 14:97–116, 1977.
37. Wright BD, Linacre JM: BIGSTEPS: Rasch Computer Program for All Two Facet Problems. Chicago, MESA Press, 1997.

38. Wright BD, Linacre JM: Observations are always ordinal: Measures, however, must be interval. Arch Phys Med Rehabil 70:857–860, 1989.
39. Wright BD, Masters GN: Rating Scale Analysis: Rasch Measurement. Chicago, MESA Press, 1982.
40. Wright BD, Stone MH: Best Test Design: Rasch Measurement. Chicago, MESA Press, 1979.

ANNE G. FISHER, ScD, OTR, FAOTA

MULTIFACETED MEASUREMENT OF DAILY LIFE TASK PERFORMANCE:

Conceptualizing a Test of Instrumental ADL and Validating the Addition of Personal ADL Tasks

From the Department of Occupational Therapy
Colorado State University
Fort Collins, Colorado

Reprint requests to:
Anne G. Fisher, ScD, OTR, FAOTA
Professor
Department of Occupational Therapy
Occupational Therapy Building
Colorado State University
Fort Collins, CO 80523

The development of a functional assessment or rehabilitation outcome measure must be guided by a clear conceptual model of the construct to be tested as well as by a sound measurement model. The conceptual model provides an operational definition of disability that is consistent with the intended purpose of the evaluation, and it guides the development of the test items and the test administration procedures. The measurement model provides a set of assertions against which the data can be evaluated to ensure that a valid measure is being constructed.

This chapter describes how we have used a conceptual model and a many-faceted Rasch measurement model to guide the development of the Assessment of Motor and Process Skills (AMPS),[10] specifically the addition of seven new personal activities of daily living (PADL) tasks to the AMPS. Following a description of the AMPS is a summary of the conceptual model and the many-faceted Rasch model that have guided the development of the AMPS. Finally, issues are discussed that we considered in the decision to add PADL tasks to the AMPS, and results of a pilot study designed to evaluate the validity of their addition to the AMPS are reported.

ASSESSMENT OF MOTOR AND PROCESS SKILLS

The AMPS is an evaluation designed to measure a person's quality of performance of domestic or instrumental activities of daily living

(IADL). The quality of performance is measured in terms of the efficiency, effectiveness, safety, or difficulty of component actions that the person uses to effect IADL task performance.

More specifically, the occupational therapist uses the AMPS to evaluate two domains of occupational performance: IADL motor skills and IADL process skills. IADL motor skills are the component actions the person uses during the performance of IADL tasks to move the task objects or themselves. IADL process skills are the actions of performance that reflect the person's ability to logically sequence the actions of the IADL task performance over time, select and use appropriate tools and materials, and adapt his or her performance when problems are encountered. The occupational therapist administers the AMPS to determine whether a person has the necessary motor and process skills to effectively, efficiently, and safely perform the IADL tasks needed for community living.

The motor and process skills shown in Table 1 are universal component actions that comprise and support all IADL task performances. For example, whether a person makes a sandwich, folds a basket of laundry, or sweeps the floor, he or she must reach for, grip, and lift the task objects. Similarly, he or she must search for and locate the needed tools and materials, gather them to the workplace, and sequence the actions of the performance in a logical order.

The AMPS is a test of disability;[41] it is not designed to evaluate for the presence of motor or cognitive impairments. However, because the AMPS includes both an IADL motor scale and an IADL process scale, the AMPS has the potential to allow the therapist to evaluate the impact of underlying impairments on the quality of the component motor or process skills, and their effect on the quality, efficiency, or effectiveness of the person's IADL task performance. In addition, the AMPS process

TABLE 1. AMPS Motor and Process Skill Items

Motor Skills	Process Skills
Posture	**Energy**
Stabilizes	Paces
Aligns	Attends
Positions	**Using Knowledge**
Mobility	Chooses
Walks	Uses
Reaches	Handles
Bends	Heeds
Coordination	Inquires
Coordinates	**Temporal Organization**
Manipulates	Initiates
Flows	Continues
Strength and Effort	Sequences
Moves	Terminates
Transports	**Space and Objects**
Lifts	Searches/locates
Calibrates	Gathers
Grips	Organizes
Energy	Restores
Endures	Navigates
Paces	**Adaptation**
	Notices/responds
	Accommodates
	Adjusts
	Benefits

skills scale provides information regarding the ability of the person to overcome residual motor and cognitive impairments by learning and using alternative strategies during task performance. The occupational therapist uses this information to plan and implement interventions designed to enhance the person's occupational performance.

The AMPS is based on the premise that a person's performance is influenced by the meaningfulness of the tasks to the person who performs them.[6,24] The administration procedures of the AMPS, therefore, are designed to allow the person to choose two or three IADL tasks to perform based on their familiarity and relevance to her- or himself. Since the AMPS has been standardized internationally and cross-culturally,[2,10,20,21,28] we must recognize that task familiarity and relevance are heavily influenced by the cultural background of the person being evaluated.[28]

To meet the demand for task choices appropriate for persons from diverse backgrounds and with diverse needs and interests, 56 standardized task choices were included in the AMPS manual. Through an informal interview between the client and the rater, AMPS task choices that are matched to the abilities, needs, interests, and cultural background of the client are narrowed by the rater to a subset of four to six relevant tasks that provide the client a sufficient level of challenge. From this subset, the client chooses two or three tasks to perform.

The client performs the tasks in accordance with the task guidelines outlined in the AMPS manual.[10] The guidelines provide sufficient criteria for each task to allow for their standardization, yet they are flexible enough to allow each person to perform the tasks in his or her usual manner using the tools and materials he or she would usually use. Flexible options also allow for the diversity of methods people use cross-culturally to perform otherwise comparable tasks. For example, to brew a pot of coffee or tea, the client is free to specify if he will brew coffee or tea, and, if he chooses to brew coffee, whether he will boil the coffee, use a French press, or make the coffee in an electric coffee maker. Persons in the United Kingdom are more likely to brew tea, while persons from the United States or Sweden are more likely to brew coffee. The use of a French press may be chosen more often by a person from Europe, Australia, New Zealand, or North America, but boiled coffee tends to be unique to northern Sweden, Alaska, and parts of New Zealand. Whatever option the client chooses, the task guidelines require that the client choose and use appropriate and prechosen tools and materials, brew the coffee or tea, serve it, and restore the workspace upon completion of the task.

Once the person has chosen the tasks he will perform, and he is fully oriented to the test environment, the occupational therapist observes the client's AMP tasks performances. The therapist then scores each motor and process skill item according to the quality of each action as observed during each of the IADL task performances. There are 16 motor and 20 process skill items (see Table 1). Each skill item is scored using a four-point ordinal scale based on the quality of performance: 1 = deficit, 2 = ineffective, 3 = questionable, and 4 = competent. The scoring criteria are designed to allow the occupational therapist to consider the client's need for assistance, level of effort (difficulty), degree of efficiency, and degree of safety. The AMPS manual provides a complete description of the guidelines for scoring an AMPS observation. AMPS raters are occupational therapists who have become certified by attending a 5-day training and calibration course and using the skills to observe and score 10 additional subjects using the AMPS.

Following scoring, the AMPS rater enters the raw scores into the rater's personal copy of the AMPS computer-scoring software. The many-faceted Rasch model[27] incorporated into this software was based on the calibration values for tasks, items, and rating scale steps derived from a calibration sample of 4689 subjects.[10] The many-faceted Rasch computer program, FACETS,[26] was used to generate the calibration values. Like FACETS, the AMPS computer-scoring program converts a person's raw AMPS skill item scores into linear person ability measures that can be placed on linear motor and process IADL continua, the AMPS motor and process scales. The person ability measures, expressed as log-odds probability units (logits), are adjusted for each individual during the Rasch analysis to account for (1) skill item difficulty, (2) task challenge, and (3) rater severity.[11,13] A higher IADL motor or process ability measure indicates that the individual is more able or higher on the continuum of the AMPS motor and process scales.

The calibrated AMPS rater is able to use the AMPS computer-scoring software to generate several reports, including the following:

AMPS Summary Report. An evaluation report that summarizes the results of the AMPS observation.

AMPS Raw Scores. A table of the client's raw scores that can be used to verify the accuracy of data entry.

Graphic Report. A visual representation of the client's ability measures plotted on the AMPS motor and process scales in reference to the cutoff measures indicative of evidence of problems that affect performance. The client's motor and process ability measures for each AMPS observation are reported at the bottom of this report.

Summary of Misfitting Ratings. Alerts the examiner to item ratings that were unexpected. The report details the skill item, the task, and whether the rating was unexpectedly high or low.

CONCEPTUAL MODEL OF THE AMPS

Figure 1 schematically represents the conceptual model of the AMPS. It illuminates the complex relationship among (1) the human open system, (2) the task to be performed, (3) the environment, (4) culture, and (5) occupational performance. The conceptual model of the AMPS originally was based on the model of human occupation[24] and led to a revision of that model to incorporate concepts defined by and during our development of the AMPS.[25] In particular, the development of the AMPS culminated in significant revision of how the mind-brain-body performance subsystem and performance skills are conceptualized within the model of human occupation.[15,16]

In developing the AMPS, we asserted that functional behavior is a complex set of interactions between the person, the task, and the environment. According to Connolly and Dalgleish, "skills are practiced abilities that show deftness, dexterity, and confidence in performance; they are goal-directed actions . . . . Skill [involves] a transaction between the performer and the environment, and to understand skilled performance it is necessary to understand the nature of the organism-environment interaction with regard to the specific context and the goal in question. Skills are always jointly determined by the organism, the task, and the precise environment in which the actions take place."[3] Therefore, we developed the AMPS based on the premise that accurate determination of a person's ability to perform daily life tasks is most directly assessed through the evaluation of his or her skills (practiced abilities) observed in the context of his or her dynamic interaction with the environment during performance of a specified task.[10]

The environment provides the social and physical context for the performance. It includes the physical spaces where the task performances occurs, the tools and

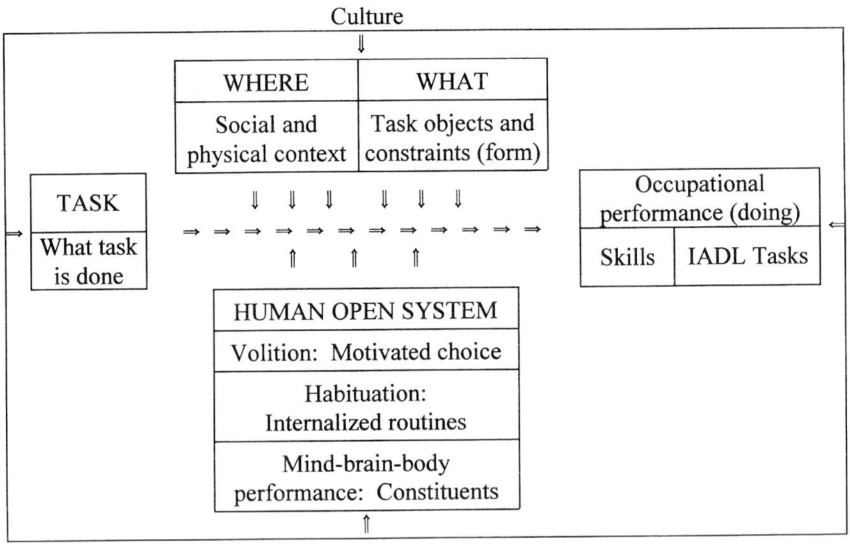

FIGURE 1. Conceptual model of the Assessment of Motor and Process Skills.

materials that are available or used, and the people who are present. Occupational forms also are derived from the environment. They are culturally defined conventions for "ways of doing" that can be named and recognized by a cultural group as being oriented to a specific purpose.[25] In the conceptual model for the AMPS, we also view occupational forms as a set of culturally defined task characteristics that result in shared recognition that "this" individual is performing "this" task. We refer to these culturally defined task characteristics as the constraints of the task, and they specify the appropriate context, the tools and materials to be used, the norms or rules for the performance, and the necessary temporal order of actions.[29]

Since occupational forms are culturally defined conventions or task characteristics, we expect that the tools and materials a person chooses to use, his or her temporal order of actions, and his or her values or norms for an expected outcome may vary somewhat from our own.[21] In the AMPS, the person must perform the tasks in a manner that would be recognized by his or her cultural group as being effective, logical, and oriented toward the goal mutually agreed upon by the person being evaluated and the rater.

Within the theoretical framework of the AMPS, we view the person being evaluated as an open system that takes in information from the environment and acts on this information to produce output in the form of occupational performance (skill and IADL task performance (see Fig. 1). We view occupational performance as a meaningful sequence of actions in which the person enacts an occupational form and completes a specified task. Performance skills are the discrete behavioral elements of performance. They are the learned motor and process skills—the component actions of performance—that are compiled to enact a form.

During an AMPS observation, what the person performs is an IADL task. It is occupation, the doing of something—the action of making a sandwich, brewing coffee, repotting a plant. The form, when named, is the accomplished task—tuna sandwich, brewed coffee, repotted plant.[12]

There is a subtle interrelationship among occupational performance (the enactment of the IADL task), the culturally shared social conventions that define the constraints of the task (form), and the task itself that is named and defined conceptually outside its actual enactment or performance. We consider the task in our conceptual model because different tasks present different levels of challenge and various tasks may be more or less familiar to the person who is being evaluated.

The evaluated person, the "human open system," comprises three interrelated subsystems that interact with each other and influence the quality of task performance. The three subsystems are volition, habituation, and the mind-brain-body performance subsystems. The volition subsystem includes dispositions and traits that guide and motivate choices for occupational performance. Volition determines "why we do what we do" and contributes to the organization of performance by giving it meaning.[10,25]

A critical component of the AMPS is our assertion that volitional (motivational) factors influence the quality of task performance. When an individual has the opportunity to choose and enter into the performance of a task that matches his or her volitional traits (i.e., value placed on the task, interest in or enjoyment derived from the task, sense of competence or belief in the ability to perform the task), task performance is maximized.[6,24] That is, the elements of the volition subsystem influence the choice to engage in task performance, and they then sustain and motivate task performance once the individual begins performing the task.

The habituation subsystem organizes "what we do" into patterns and "when we do it" into routines.[10] The components of the habituation system include organizational structures and images called role scripts and habit maps. Role scripts are internalized expectations of what it means to be and how to be someone of particular social identity and related obligations. Role scripts guide the related construction of actions that are used to enact a given role. Habit maps are internalized structures that guide well-learned patterns of behavior to helps us construct daily routines and style of doing.[25] This subsystem is primarily relevant to the logical organization of task performance over time; role scripts and habit maps are internalized models or rules that help us to organize behavior into socially recognizable patterns or routines (occupational forms). Within the context of an AMPS observation, a person who has lost or has never developed well-defined role scripts and habit maps is likely to experience disruption in the enactment of socially defined forms, the IADL tasks the person chooses to perform.

The mind-brain-body performance subsystem constitutes "what we have to do it with" and includes the structures used by the human open system to effect occupational performance. The constituents are (1) musculoskeletal, (2) neurologic, (3) cardiopulmonary, and (4) cognitive.[10,15]

Impairments[41] result when there is disruption of the mind-brain-body subsystem. Impairments include the capacity to reach, to lift, to remember, or to sequence. The AMPS is not designed to test impairments. As a test of disability, the AMPS is designed to evaluate whether the person effectively reaches for the plate from the cupboard shelf, lifts the bag of bread from the table, chooses needed tools and materials or heeds the goal of the IADL task, and performs the steps of the IADL task in a logical order. Capacities (impairments) pertain to strength, range of motion, memory, and cognition; IADL skills or abilities (disability) pertain to the quality of a person's daily life task performance.[41] The AMPS is used to evaluate whether any existing impairments have impacted learned motor and process skills such that they directly affect the quality, efficiency, or effectiveness of the person's IADL task performance.

Finally, culture (shared beliefs, values, and customs) influences where we perform tasks, what tasks we do, how we do them, and what tools and materials we use.[21,28] Culture also plays an important role in the development of internalized values and internalized role scripts and habit maps.[25] The conceptual model of the AMPS recognizes the pervasive role of culture in occupational performance, an important requirement for an assessment tool designed for international, cross-cultural applications that ensures valid measurement within a context where the evaluated person performs familiar, culture-relevant IADL tasks of his or her choosing.[2,20,21,28]

THE AMPS MANY-FACETED MEASUREMENT MODEL

With the conceptual model serving as a guide, we developed the AMPS in response to the need for a valid and reliable assessment that allows for the individual's choice of specific IADL tasks and describes the quality of a person's IADL task performance in a manner that can be used to guide treatment planning. This required that we use a measurement model that allowed us to calibrate and equate tasks for their challenges, discover the hierarchical order of the AMPS skill item difficulties and the task challenges, and verify that the skill items and tasks work together to define unidimensional constructs.[11,13,14]

The AMPS IADL tasks vary from simple to complex, and each is conceptualized as the outcome of a series of actions that can be observed as the person compiles them to effect task performance. For the AMPS, we identified two taxonomies of actions that could be observed across all IADL task performances (see Table 1); actions that were not universal were eliminated in the early phases of the development of the AMPS.

Each client assessment is based on observing the person perform at least two IADL tasks that are of sufficient challenge to ensure reasonable, if not ideal, item targeting. Each set of tasks that compose a client assessment can be considered a different test or "version" of the AMPS. All possible versions of the AMPS are contained in a large item bank.

Wright reports, "Data from different tasks taken by different candidates can be combined and analyzed together, so long as there is some network of commonalities (candidates and/or items) linking the tests . . . . Once a bank of items has been calibrated, inclusion of items from the bank into each new test automatically equates that test to the common metric of the bank, as so to all other tests derived from the bank."[42] Through a process of gathering data on thousands of linked AMPS task observations, we have constructed a large item bank for a functional assessment composed of two scales, an IADL motor scale and an IADL process scale. More specifically, each AMPS scale has a total of 56 tasks. Each task is associated with the 16 common or universal motor items and the 20 common or universal process items. Hence, the AMPS can be considered an item bank that contains 896 motor items and 1120 process items. Each client assessment, based on observing the client perform at least two AMPS tasks, is composed of a subset of at least 32 motor items and 40 process items available in the entire AMPS item bank.

Equating of AMPS tasks, linked by common skill items, makes it possible to compare the ability of a client who performed one set of tasks upon initial evaluation with the results of his performance on a different set of tasks upon reevaluation. Similarly, equating allows performance to be compared among several clients who each performed a different set of AMPS tasks.

The AMPS was developed to meet the need for unidimensional, linear scales that permit the simultaneous assessment of two universal sets of discrete performance skills and the interdependence of these motor and process skills in IADL task performance. The AMPS motor and process skill items and 56 IADL tasks, therefore, all had to be calibrated on two common linear scales (IADL motor scale and IADL process scale) based on the relative difficulty of the skill items and the relative challenge of the tasks.

Because raters needed to be calibrated for their relative severities when scoring the skill items on each AMPS scale, severity was calibrated on the same common linear scale. This need to calibrate tasks, items, and raters on common linear scales required that we use a many-faceted Rasch model[27] to develop the AMPS. By calibrating the severity of the raters, the challenge of the tasks, and the difficulty of the skills items on the same linear scales, we can obtain person IADL motor and IADL process ability measures that are adjusted for severity of the raters and the challenge of the tasks actually performed.[11,13]

The many-faceted Rasch model used for the AMPS is based on the assertions that:

- A person is more likely to obtain a higher score on an easy skill item than on a hard skill item,
- Easy skill items are more likely to be easier for all persons than are hard skill items,
- Raters are more likely to award higher scores for easy skill items than for hard skill items,
- Lenient raters are more likely to award higher scores to all persons than are severe raters,
- All persons are more likely to obtain higher scores on simple tasks than on complex tasks, and
- Persons with higher ability are more likely to score higher overall than are persons with lower ability.[10,11,13]

Ever since our first application of the FACETS many-faceted Rasch analysis computer program[26] to our data a decade ago, we have continually monitored our data to ensure that the AMPS tasks, the motor and process skill items, and the AMPS raters work together to define two unidimensional scales. Our criteria for unidimensionality have been based on goodness of fit to the many faceted Rasch model.

Data from more than 12,000 people from North America, Scandinavia, the United Kingdom, Australia, New Zealand, Holland, Israel, and Asia have been entered into the AMPS database. The 56 tasks and 36 skill items have been shown to fit the measurement model (infit and outfit mean square [MnSq] values ≤ 1.4 and ≥ 0.6 associated with $t < 2$ or > -2). High inter- and intrarater reliability exists among the more than 900 calibrated raters. That is, the overall rate of misfit of individual AMPS skill item ratings remains close to expected values (motor: 1.0% at $t \geq 3$ or ≤ -3 process: 0.9% at $t \geq 3$ or ≤ -3). Moreover, 97% of the raters demonstrate goodness-of-fit statistics indicative of consistent scoring according to the assertions of the measurement model. Among the 4689 subjects used to estimate the calibration values used in the AMPS computer-scoring program, 94% demonstrated fit to the model for the AMPS motor scale and 95% demonstrated fit to the model for the AMPS process scale.

ADDITION OF PADL TASKS TO THE AMPS

Our original goal in the development of the AMPS was to find a tool that could be applied equally to all populations without regard for age (5–100 years), diagnosis, degree of motor or cognitive ability, or culture or region of residence. This required the construction of linear scales of sufficient length to allow testing of low-functioning persons as well as those who are more able and live independently in the community. Our intention was to design the AMPS to minimize the problems of tools that lack sensitivity at the upper and lower ends of the scale.

AMPS raters recently have suggested that there may be a need to extend the range of the AMPS scales down to include easier tasks that enable us to evaluate clients who are too disabled or frail, too young, or who have no need or interest in doing IADL tasks.

We originally did not include personal ADL tasks in the AMPS because numerous tests of PADL already existed and PADL and IADL may represent two different constructs.[10] Several advantages of the AMPS, however, led to our recognition that adding PADL tasks to the AMPS had the potential to meet existing needs beyond those realized merely by extending the range of the AMPS scales.

While Fisher, Harvey, and Kilgore argued against the "massive proliferation" functional status instruments, they also recognized that "different applications require different degrees of specificity, precision, and accuracy, and they may well also require different ranges in the measurement continuum."[17] The AMPS is not like most existing functional status instruments designed to measure activities of daily living.

Most global scales of ADL emphasize the physical or motor component of ADL task performance, expressed in terms of independence or need for assistance.[37,38,43] Reuben has expressed concern that such scales are insensitive to change.[34] Moreover, Reuben reports that "most of the scales developed have created response categories that indicate the degree of assistance required, which, albeit important, frame disability in economic terms (i.e., resource demand) rather than personal estimates of quality of life. More recently developed scales . . . have phrased responses in terms of degree of difficulty and amount of limitation. One can argue the pros and cons of each approach, but clearly none is comprehensive. Moreover, the differences in how functional status questions are phrased are not trivial."[34]

In most existing tests of ADL, the test items ("questions") are global, referring to behaviors such as upper body dressing, meal preparation, or home management, which are scored based on level of assistance needed (what can the person do). In contrast, the AMPS test items are the component motor and process actions of the task performance (see Table 1). The scoring criteria for each AMPS skill item have been designed such that the rater considers not only need for assistance but also the quality of the performance as indicated by level of effort, degree of efficiency, and safety of the performance. The result is a broader and more detailed view of what the person can do effectively, and why a person may experience problems in ADL task performance.

In the AMPS, there are a variety of IADL tasks options within an area that commonly is considered as only one or two items on a global ADL scale. Rather than score the person on all items regardless of their relevance to the person, the AMPS allows the person to perform tasks that are relevant to his or her daily needs. The rater then scores quality of the person's IADL motor and process skills in the context of task performances that are meaningful to the person being evaluated. The result is *client-centered assessment*, a term that refers to evaluation procedures that are individualized and sensitive to the person's varying needs, interests, and contexts.[33]

While we are aware that scales that include both PADL and IADL have the potential to better identify problems in daily life task performance and need for service,[39] our concern was whether PADL and IADL ability were one construct or two.

TABLE 4. Goodness-of-Fit for the PADL Tasks

Task	Infit MnSq	Infit t	Outfit MnSq	Outfit t
Motor				
Eating a meal	1.1	0	1.1	0
Brushing teeth	0.9	0	0.9	0
Upper body grooming/bathing	1.0	0	0.9	0
Putting on socks/shoes—slip-on	1.0	0	1.1	0
Putting on socks/shoes—tied	0.9	−2	0.9	−1
Upper body dressing	1.0	0	1.0	0
Upper/lower body dressing	0.9	0	1.0	0
Process				
Eating a meal	0.9	−1	0.9	0
Brushing teeth	0.7	−3	0.7	−3
Upper body grooming/bathing	0.8	−5	0.8	−4
Putting on socks/shoes—slip-on	0.7	−3	0.7	−3
Putting on socks/shoes—tied	0.8	−4	0.7	−3
Upper body dressing	0.8	−3	0.8	−3
Upper/lower body dressing	1.0	0	0.9	0

PADL tasks. We can infer this because (1) a person is more likely to obtain a higher score on an easy skill item than on a hard skill item and (2) easy skill items are more likely to be easier for all persons than are hard skill items regardless of whether the person performed IADL or PADL tasks. Otherwise, the tasks would not demonstrate acceptable fit for the IADL-based model. While direct comparison of separately estimated motor and process skill item hierarchies for only the IADL tasks vs. only the PADL tasks will be needed to verify these conclusions, the present results do support the universality of the AMPS skill items.

For three of the PADL tasks, we had sufficient data to ensure reasonably stable task challenge calibrations (Table 5). Overall, these three PADL tasks (upper body

TABLE 5. AMPS Motor and Process Task Simplicity Calibration Values—Selected Tasks (Logits)

	Motor			Process		
Easy	0.68	Upper body dressing	⇐	1.07	Shoes and socks: tied	⇐
	0.60	Upper body grooming/bathing	⇐	1.03	Upper body dressing	⇐
	0.46	Shoes and socks: tied	⇐	0.82	Cold drink from refrigerator	
	0.38	Machine wash laundry		0.64	Make standard bed	
	0.37	Cold drink from refrigerator		0.54	Machine wash laundry	
	0.37	Hot or cold instant drink		0.53	Fold laundry	
	0.35	Fold laundry		0.50	Upper body grooming/bathing	⇐
	0.29	Wash dishes		0.43	Hot or cold instant drink	
	0.25	Cottage cheese and fruit salad		0.39	Make Swedish bed	
	0.16	Set table		0.36	Hand wash laundry	
	0.15	Hand wash laundry		0.30	Polish shoes	
	0.15	Ironing: No set-up required		0.29	Fried ripe plátanos	
	⋮			⋮		
	−0.23	Mop floor		−0.48	Eggs, meat, and brewed coffee	
	−0.24	French toast and beverage		−0.50	Omelette, toast, and beverage	
	−0.27	Change Swedish style bed		−0.56	Eggs, toast, and brewed coffee	
	−0.31	Vacuum		−0.70	French toast and beverage	
Hard	−0.35	Eggs, toast, and Cuban coffee		−0.78	Eggs, toast, and Cuban coffee	

Arrows refer to new PADL tests.

dressing, upper body grooming/bathing, and putting on shoes and socks—fastened or tied) were easier than the IADL tasks. The new PADL tasks extended the range of both AMPS scales by about 0.20 logits. The effective range of the AMPS process scale remains greater than that of the AMPS motor scale.

More importantly, the addition of PADL tasks offers more options for persons who are not able or who have little interest in performing IADL tasks. While there is often a perception among therapists who take AMPS training and calibration courses that men, in particular, do not perform IADL tasks, the problems of finding AMPS IADL tasks that are familiar, relevant, and appropriately challenging for men is rarely a problem in practice. However, persons who are frail or confined to bed cannot perform many of the IADL tasks, persons who live in nursing homes often no longer want to or are not allowed to perform IADL tasks, or children who are younger than 5 or 6 often have not yet learned to perform many of the AMPS IADL tasks. Our addition of PADL tasks to the AMPS extends the usefulness of the AMPS to these individuals.

An important feature of the AMPS is that the client has the opportunity to choose the tasks he or she will perform. However, the choices of tasks offered to the client are limited by the examiner to ones that offer an appropriate level of challenge. Because the PADL tasks tend to be easier than the IADL tasks, the examiner must restrict the use of the PADL tasks to frail adults or young children. When more able clients are allowed to perform IADL or PADL tasks that are too easy, greater error in estimating the person ability measures is introduced due to the off-targeting of the AMPS skill items relative to the ability of the person tested.

CONCLUSION

A conceptual model defines *what* is to be measured and *how* it is to be measured. In the AMPS, we view occupational performance—an interaction between the person, the task, and the environment—as being influenced by culture and individual choice. The performance is a series of universal motor and process skills that are compiled to enact an occupational form. Using this model as a guide, we identified tasks, items, and administration procedures that were consistent with our model. Then we used a many-faceted Rasch model to monitor and evaluate the data to ensure that we were constructing a valid, reliable, unidimensional measure.

The choice of items to include in most ADL tests has been driven by "item content specification" derived from expert opinion and common practice. Because this approach does not ensure that the test is testing the intended construct,[13] we chose a different approach to item selection. We began with a conceptual model and allowed the model to drive the design and content of the AMPS. We then verified our conceptual model through determination that the data conformed to the assertions of the many-faceted Rasch model and measured two unidimensional constructs.

Future research will focus on gathering more data, reevaluating the fit of all of the PADL tasks to the many-faceted Rasch model for the AMPS that has been defined by the IADL tasks, examining the hierarchal order of the PADL tasks among themselves and among the IADL tasks, and evaluating the stability of the item difficulty hierarchies between the IADL tasks and the new PADL tasks. As we consider the addition of new tasks to the AMPS system, either to increase the range of the scales or to offer a greater variety of task options, we will continue to select tasks based on their theoretical fit to our conceptual model and validate them via many-faceted Rasch analyses for statistical fit to the assertions of the AMPS measurement model.

ACKNOWLEDGMENT

This chapter is based on a presentation given at the MESA Psychometric Laboratory–Rehabilitation Foundation Inc. Invitational Conference on Outcome Measurement in Rehabilitation, May 31, 1996, at the University of Chicago. It was supported in part by grant RO1-AG12345-03, Development of a Performance Evaluation for Gerontology, by the National Institute on Aging, National Institutes of Health, U.S. Department of Health and Human Services. The author's appreciation is extended to Bradley Atchison, Birgitta Bernspång, Leslie Duran, Karen Kirkley, and Julie Gibbs Long for their reviews and critical feedback on earlier versions of this manuscript.

REFERENCES

1. Bernspång B, Fisher AG: Differences between persons with right or left CVA on the Assessment of Motor and Process Skills. Arch Phys Med Rehabil 76:1144–1151, 1995.
2. Bernspång B, Fisher AG: Validation of the Assessment of Motor and Process Skills for use in Sweden. Scand J Occup Ther 2:3–9, 1995.
3. Connolly K, Dalgleish M: The emergence of a tool-using skill in infancy. Dev Psychol 25:894–912, 1989.
4. Dickerson AE, Fisher AG: Age differences in functional performance. Am J Occup Ther 47:686–692, 1993.
5. Dickerson AE, Fisher AG: Culture-relevant functional performance assessment of the Hispanic elderly. Occup Ther J Res 15:50–68, 1995.
6. Doble S: Intrinsic motivation and clinical practice: The key to understanding the unmotivated client. Can J Occup Ther 55:75–81, 1988.
7. Doble SE, Fisk JD, Fisher AG, et al: Functional competence of community-dwelling persons with multiple sclerosis using the Assessment of Motor and Process Skills. Arch Phys Med Rehabil 75:843–851, 1994.
8. Duran L, Fisher AG: A comparison of male and female performance of the Assessment of Motor and Process Skills. Arch Phys Med Rehabil 77:1019–1024, 1996.
9. Finch M, Kane RL, Philp I: Developing a new metric for ADLs. J Am Geriatr Soc 43:877–884, 1995.
10. Fisher AG: Assessment of Motor and Process Skills (rev. ed.). Fort Collins, CO, Three Star Press, 1995.
11. Fisher AG: Development of a functional assessment that adjusts ability measures for task simplicity and rater leniency. In Wilson M (ed): Objective Measurement: Theory into Practice. Vol 2. Norwood, NJ, Ablex, 1994, pp 145–175.
12. Fisher AG: Functional assessment and occupation: Critical issues for occupational therapy. N Z J Occup Ther 45(2):13–19, 1994.
13. Fisher AG: The assessment of IADL motor skills: An application of many faceted Rasch analysis. Am J Occup Ther 47:319–329, 1993.
14. Fisher AG, Bryze KA, Granger CV, et al: Applications of Rasch analysis to the development of functional measures. Int J Educ Res 21:579–593, 1994.
15. Fisher AG, Kielhofner G: Mind-brain-body performance subsystem. In Kielhofner G (ed): A Model of Human Occupation: Theory and Application. 2nd ed. Baltimore, Williams & Wilkins, 1995, pp 83–89.
16. Fisher AG, Kielhofner G: Skill in occupational performance. In Kielhofner G (ed): A Model of Human Occupation: Theory and Application. 2nd ed. Baltimore,Williams & Wilkins, 1995, pp 113–137.
17. Fisher WP, Harvey RF, Kilgore KM: New developments in functional assessment: Probabilistic models for gold standards. Neurorehabilitation 5:3–25, 1995.
18. Folstein MF, Folstein SE, McHugh PR: Mini-Mental State: A practical method for grading the cognitive state of patients for the clinician. J Psychiatr Res 12:189–198, 1975.
19. Girard CR, Fisher AG, Short MS: Daily life performance differences between psychiatric groups [manuscript].
20. Goldman SL, Fisher AG: Validation of the cross-cultural universality of the Assessment of Motor and Process Skills 60:77–85, 1997.
21. Goto S, Fisher AG, Mayberry WL: AMPS applied cross-culturally to the Japanese. Am J Occup Ther 50:798–806, 1996.
22. Keith RA, Granger CV, Hamilton BB, Sherwin FS: The Functional Independence Measure: A new tool for rehabilitation. In Eisenberg NG, Grzesiak RC (eds): Advances in Clinical Rehabilitation. Vol 1. New York, Springer-Verlag, 1987, pp 6–18.

23. Kempen GIJM, Suurmeijer TPBM: The development of a hierarchical polychotomous ADL-IADL scale for noninstitutionalized elders. Gerontologist 30:497–502, 1990.
24. Kielhofner G: A Model of Human Occupation: Theory and Application. Baltimore, Williams & Wilkins, 1985.
25. Kielhofner G: A Model of Human Occupation: Theory and Applications. 2nd ed. Baltimore, Williams & Wilkins, 1995.
26. Linacre JM: Facets: Many-facet Rasch Measurement Computer Program. Chicago, MESA Press, 1987–1994.
27. Linacre JM: Many-facet Rasch Measurements. 2nd ed. Chicago, MESA Press, 1993.
28. Magalhães L, Fisher AG, Bernspång B, Linacre JM: Cross-cultural assessment of functional ability. Occup Ther J Res 16:45–63, 1996.
29. Nelson D: Occupation: Form and performance. Am J Occup Ther 42:633–641, 1988.
30. Nygård L, Bernspång B, Fisher AG, Winblad B: Comparing motor and process ability of persons with suspected dementia in home and clinic settings. Am J Occup Ther 48:689–696, 1994.
31. Pan AW, Fisher AG: The Assessment of Motor and Process Skills of persons with psychiatric disorders. Am J Occup Ther 48:775–780, 1994 .
32. Park S, Fisher AG, Velozo CA: Using the Assessment of Motor and Process Skills to compare occupational performance between clinic and home settings. Am J Occup Ther 48:697–709, 1994.
33. Pollock N: Client-centered assessment. Am J Occup Ther 47:298–301, 1993.
34. Reuben DB: What's wrong with ADLs? J Am Geriatr Soc 43:936–937, 1995.
35. Robinson S, Fisher AG: A study to examine the relationship of the Assessment of Motor and Process Skills (AMPS) to other tests of cognition and function. Br J Occup Ther 59:260–263, 1996.
36. Roth M, Mountjoy CQ, Huppert FA, et al: CAMDEX: The Cambridge Examination for Mental Disorders of the Elderly. Cambridge, England, Cambridge University Press, 1986.
37. Silverstein B, Fisher WP, Kilgore KM, et al: Applying psychometric criteria to functional assessment in medical rehabilitation. II: Defining interval measures. Arch Phys Med Rehabil 73:493–515, 1992.
38. Siu AL, Reuben DB, Hays RD: Hierarchical measures of physical function in ambulatory geriatrics. J Am Geriatr Soc 38:1113–1119, 1990.
39. Spector WD, Katz S, Murphy JB, Fulton JP: The hierarchical relationship between activities of daily living and instrumental activities of daily living. J Chron Dis 40:481–489, 1987.
40. Suurmeijer TPBM, Doeglas DM, Mown T, et al: The Groningen activity restriction scale for measuring disability: Its utility in international comparisons. Am J Public Health 84:1270–1273, 1994.
41. World Health Organization: International Classification of Impairments, Disabilities, and Handicaps. Geneva, WHO, 1980.
42. Wright B: Equitable test equating. Rasch Measure Trans 7:298–299, 1993.
43. Wright BD, Linacre JM, Heinemann AW: Measuring functional status in rehabilitation. Phys Med Rehabil Clin North Am 4:475–491, 1993.

JOHN G. BAKER, PHD
CARL V. GRANGER, MD

APPLICATION OF RASCH ANALYSIS IN THE DEVELOPMENT OF THE MEDICAL REHABILITATION FOLLOW ALONG MEASURE (MRFA)

From the Center for Functional Assessment Research
Department of Rehabilitation Medicine
State University of New York at Buffalo
Buffalo, New York

Reprint requests to:
John G. Baker, PhD
Center for Functional Assessment Research
232 Parker Hall
State University of New York at Buffalo
Buffalo, NY 14214

Quality of daily living can be thought of as a balance between the demands of a person's everyday environment and the resources or strategies that he or she uses to deal with functional limitations to achieve satisfying performance. In an outpatient setting, measuring several dimensions of this person-environment interaction allows for a more comprehensive assessment of an individual's day-to-day functioning. The quality of daily living among persons living in the community and receiving outpatient rehabilitation treatment can be considered in terms of physical, emotional, and social or role dimensions. Pain, cognitive limitations, and satisfaction are other aspects of quality of daily living.

While a multidimensional perspective is important in the development of an outpatient functional assessment measure, consistency in assessing each of the individual dimensions is essential to an accurate and reproducible measure. Frequent repeated assessments are often necessary to identify changes in functioning for persons living in the community. Thus, the accuracy with which changes in each dimension can be measured is important for the generalizability of the dimensions to overall quality of daily living.

Rasch analysis provides a methodology to develop a unidimensional, linear measure from a set of items that are considered to assess a particular aspect or dimension of outpatient daily functioning. This chapter describes the development, using Rasch analysis, of an outpatient functional assessment measure, the Medical Rehabilitation Follow Along (MRFA). The musculoskeletal form of the MRFA is used in this description. This illustration of the application of Rasch analysis provides insights into several salient issues in outpatient functional assessment. As is often the case with the application of Rasch techniques, the measurement methodology helps to elucidate aspects of the phenomenon being measured.

THE MEDICAL REHABILITATION FOLLOW ALONG MEASURES

The development of the Medical Rehabilitation Follow Along Measures has been discussed in recent studies of reliability and validity[1,2,6] and is summarized later in this chapter. The MRFA is designed to assist in screening and outcome assessment and to monitor progress in outpatient rehabilitation treatment. Currently, forms are available for musculoskeletal and neurologic problems and for multiple sclerosis. The musculoskeletal form of the MRFA has scales that assess three domains: physical functioning, the experience of pain, and affective well-being. It includes major concepts from the Functional Assessment Screening Questionnaire,[8] the Oswestry Scale,[5] and the short form of the McGill Pain Questionnaire.[11] The Brief Symptom Inventory[4] formed a basis for development originally, with subsequent revision of the items.

Domains of the MRFA

The physical functioning domain of the musculoskeletal form includes several components.[6] In part I, four general areas of functioning (personal care, lifting, walking, and traveling) are rated using six levels of functioning with specific descriptions for each level. In part II, six items describing specific tasks are rated by the respondent according to the degree of difficulty in performing each of the tasks. Together, these items make up a scale called Body Movement and Control (BMC). The early version of part I of the BMC was developed as a screening and outcome assessment tool for rehabilitation patients in primary care settings. The tasks were designed to identify problems in functioning early and to provide clues to impairment of particular organ systems.[7,8] The BMC scale of the MRFA was developed to reflect relationships, in both a diagnostic and prescriptive sense, between particular activities and the body segments or dynamics involved in the activity. An additional single effort item in the physical functioning domain asks about the patient's perception of his or her ability to exert effort in terms of strenuous physical activity. This item asks the patient to rate, on a six-point scale, the most strenuous level of physical activity that he or she can do for at least 2 minutes.

The second domain of the MRFA musculoskeletal form focuses on the experience of pain and was developed from a Rasch analysis of the short form McGill Pain Questionnaire. It includes six descriptive pain words rated by the patient as none, mild, moderate, or severe. These items clarify perception of recent pain over the past three days. Four additional descriptive pain words also are rated. A separate pain item involves a visual analog rating scale. The visual analog pain scale is marked by the patient and provides an assessment of the intensity of recent pain.

The third domain of the MRFA musculoskeletal form includes seven items that inquire about how much the person is bothered or worried in association with particular feelings and thoughts, including feelings of loneliness or being uptight. These items assess the degree of affective distress usually associated with anxiety and depression. An additional single item in the affective domain assesses satisfaction with life in general. This satisfaction item rates overall life satisfaction as very satisfied, fairly well satisfied, more satisfied than not, or not satisfied. The response can be reflective of situational tone and may relate to the patient's health condition or areas of the person's life such as a job or family situation.

Development and Scaling Using Rasch Analysis

Responses from the original 24-item Functional Assessment Screening Questionnaire (FASQ) for approximately 750 subjects with musculoskeletal problems were compiled along with responses from the Oswestry Scale, the short form McGill Pain Questionnaire, and the items describing affective distress.[6] The data were analyzed using Rasch modeling techniques with the BIGSTEPS computer program[10] to develop linear measures.

The BIGSTEPS program uses log-odd measurement units called logits to calibrate item difficulty and measure subject ability on the same scale with equal interval characteristics. The program employs fit statistics to identify how well the scale items and the persons being assessed fit the model of a linear measure. The product of the Rasch analysis is a conversion of a raw-score, nonlinear scale into a measure with unidimensionality and additivity. Responses to the various items in the measure can thus be compared along a single metric. The goal of the Rasch analysis is to produce a measure that functions on an interval level with good clinical precision (reliability) and acceptable fit characteristics (quantitative validity). Identification of items that are most useful for a scale decreases redundancy and respondent burden.

The measures for the three domains of the musculoskeletal MRFA that resulted from the Rasch analysis have been described above. The BMC measure in the physical functioning domain illustrates the application of Rasch analysis in developing a measure. The BMC measure was developed to reflect the relationships between particular types of tasks or activities and the body segments or dynamics involved in

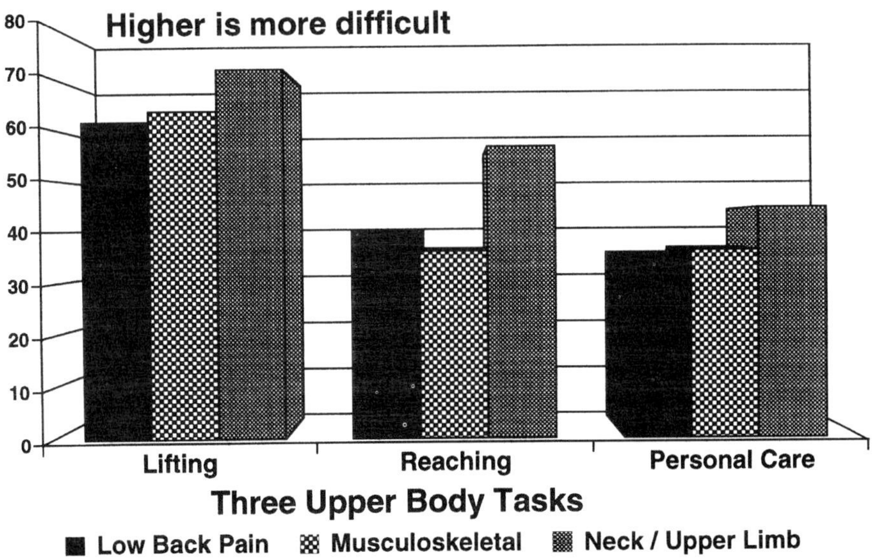

FIGURE 1. Item logit values for three upper body tasks.

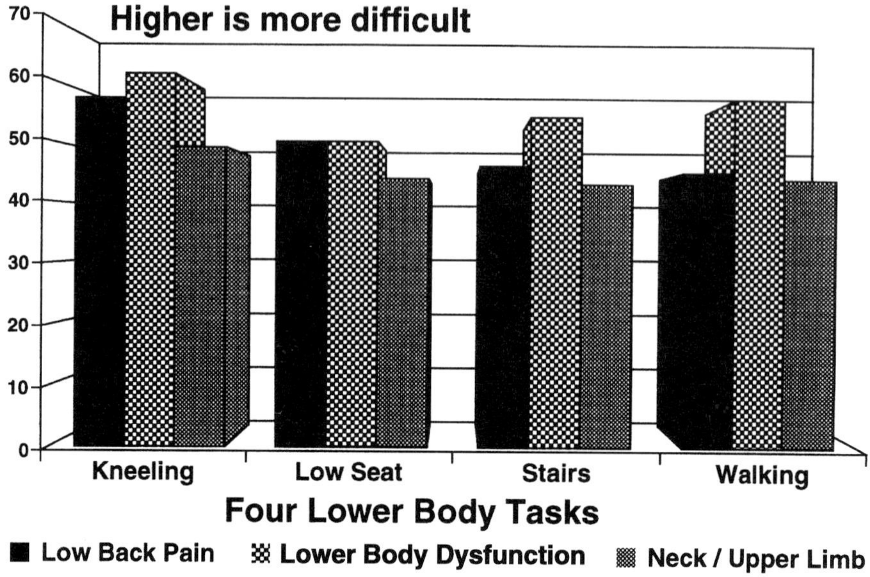

FIGURE 2. Item logit values for four lower body tasks.

the activity. The relative difficulties for the tasks or activities, in terms of their Rasch item logit values, are illustrated for different kinds of musculoskeletal problems in Figures 1–3. Figure 1 presents upper body motions reflected in the items that assess lifting, reaching, and performing personal care. Figure 2 presents lower body motions reflected in walking, stair climbing, getting up from a low seat, and kneeling

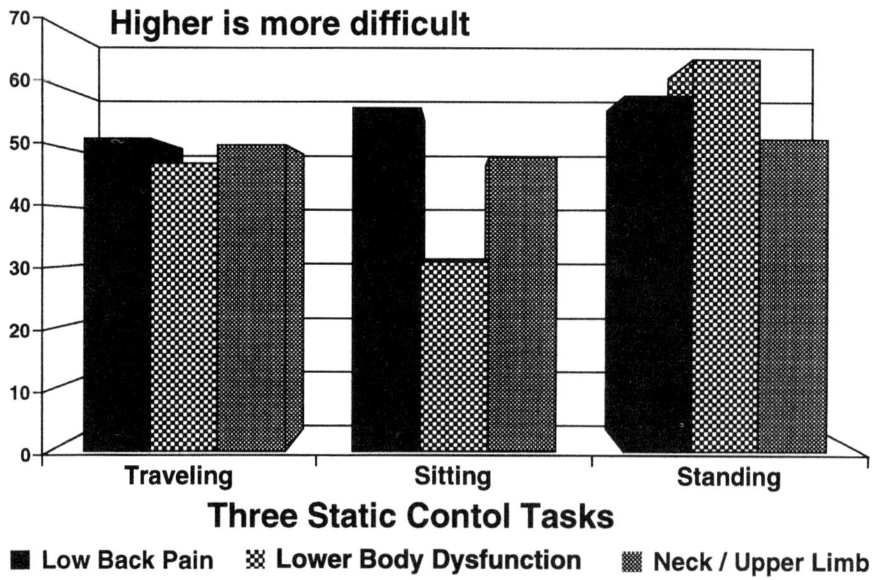

FIGURE 3. Logit values for three static control tasks.

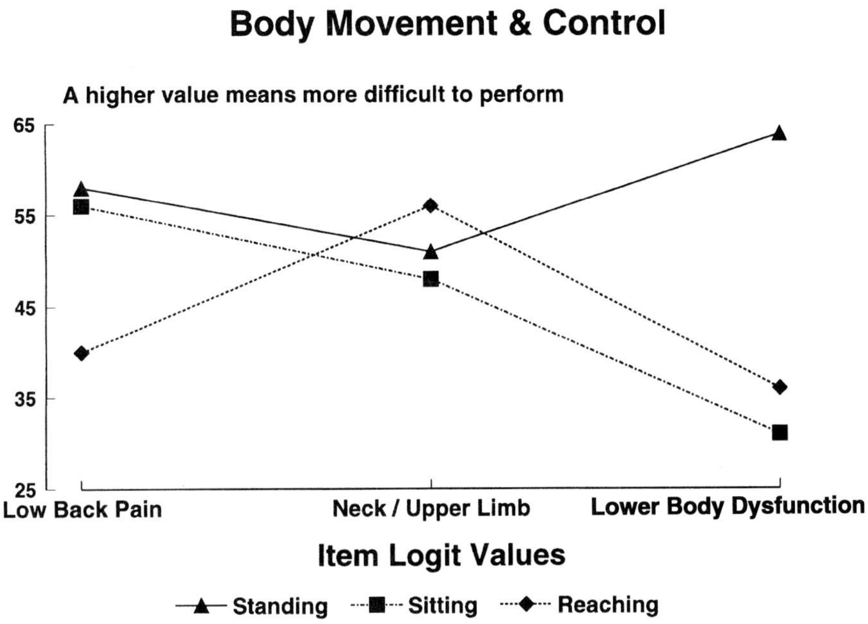

FIGURE 4. Summary of three tasks with three types of musculoskeletal problems.

and bending. Static control, reflected in items that assess sitting for 30 minutes, standing for 30 minutes, and traveling in an automobile, is illustrated in Figure 3. The figures illustrate that items representing upper body, lower body, and static control activities show different difficulties for persons with various musculoskeletal problems.

Through an analysis of function in a diagnostic sense, capabilities reflected in the three types of tasks or activities may be identified for therapeutic strengthening or for other interventions to help with appropriate adaptation. Figure 4 summarizes this diagnostic utility using three of the ten items from the BMC measure; it shows that items assessing static sitting and standing (based on average item logit values) are relatively more difficult than reaching at eye level for a person with low back pain. For someone with neck pain or upper limb dysfunction, reaching at eye level is relatively more difficult than for someone with low back pain or lower body dysfunction. For a person with lower body dysfunction, such as a gait difficulty due to an orthopedic or neurologic disorder, static standing is more difficult than sitting or reaching.

Reliability of the MRFA

The test-retest reliability of the MRFA musculoskeletal form was investigated with a sample of 47 patients receiving services at a spine and rehabilitation outpatient clinic.[6] Participants completed the MRFA at their clinic visit and again at home several days later. Responses were compared using intraclass and kappa correlation coefficients. In the physical functioning domain, ICC values ranged from 0.74 for personal care to 0.97 for driving (overall ICC = 0.83). ICC values for the items in the pain measure ranged from 0.73 to 0.84. In the affective well-being domain, ICC values ranged from 0.75 to 0.93, except for the terror/panic item, which showed an ICC of 0.44 (this item is being studied further). The pattern of kappa values was similar to those obtained for the ICC coefficients. Overall, the results of this investigation demonstrated that the musculoskeletal form of the MRFA Rasch measure produced good test-retest reliability with this sample of rehabilitation outpatients.

Validity of the MRFA

The validity of inferences made from the Rasch measures for the physical functioning, pain experience, and affective well-being domains of the MRFA was investigated with a different sample of outpatients at the spine and rehabilitation clinic.[1,2] At their initial clinic visit, 94 patients completed the musculoskeletal form of the MRFA measure along with the Medical Outcomes Trust SF-36.[13] At the completion of their outpatient rehabilitation program, participants again completed the MRFA and SF-36. The SF-36 has eight scales, including physical functioning (PF) and mental health (MH), which correspond to the Body Movement and Control (BMC) and Placid measures of the MRFA, respectively. The reliability and validity of the SF-36 has been established in numerous studies. For the present study, Rasch measures were developed for the PF and MH scales of the SF-36 using the initial assessment sample of 94 patients. Previous studies have described Rasch analyses of the PF scale of the SF-36.[9]

Content validity of the MRFA was supported by the Rasch analyses described above, which resulted in unidimensional, linear measures. As an illustration, Rasch measures and INFIT/OUTFIT statistics are presented in Table 1 for the BMC items with a sample of persons with low back pain. The Rasch measures demonstrate good item separation and INFIT/OUTFIT statistics that are within ±2.0.

Rasch Measures Before and After Rehabilitation

The construct validity for the MRFA was investigated in several ways. First, the patterns of initial Rasch measures and change in Rasch measures for the BMC and Placid measures of the MRFA were compared to the PF and MH measures of

TABLE 1. Rasch Item Measures and INFIT/OUTFIT statistics for Persons with Low Back Pain (N = 48)

Medical Rehabilitation Follow Along (Body Movement and Control)		
BMC Item	*Rasch Item Measures*	*INFIT/OUTFIT Statistic*
1. Lift (UB)	61	–1.3/–1.2
2. Kneel (LB)	57	0.5/0.4
3. Stand (SC)	56	0.8/0.8
4. Sit (SC)	56	–0.1/–0.2
5. Travel (SC)	53	–0.6/–0.6
6. Low seat (LB)	51	–1.8/–1.9
7. Walk (LB)	50	0.4/0.8
8. Stairs (LB)	45	0.9/0.9
9. Personal (UB)	38	–1.4/–0.9
10. Reach (UB)	32	0.9/0.8

(UB): Assesses primarily upper body dynamics
(LB): Assesses primarily lower body dynamics
(SC): Assesses static equilibrium and control

the SF-36. The physical (PCS) and mental (MCS) component summary scales of the SF-36, which are norm-referenced to the United States population, were used as a reference for the initial values of the MRFA and SF-36 Rasch measures. On the component summary scales, the sample showed substantially decreased initial physical functioning and about average initial emotional functioning. The initial BMC and Placid Rasch measures of the MRFA reflected this difference in physical and emotional functioning. The PF and MH Rasch measures of the SF-36 showed the same pattern.

The pattern of the change in Rasch measures from before to after rehabilitation also was comparable for the MRFA and SF-36 measures. The value of percent of initial standard deviation was used to determine change. Generally, the Rasch measures indicated that the percent of initial standard deviation value for physical functioning improved considerably as a result of physical therapy (BMC +95%, PF +77%), whereas affective state showed much less change (Placid +24%, MH +13%). As a result of the physical therapy intervention, the percent of initial standard deviation value of the Painfree measure of the MRFA improved about 82%. The pain measure of the MRFA is not directly comparable to that of the SF-36. Another measure of pain and disability called "Backill," which was developed specifically for persons with low back pain using Rasch analysis,[12] showed an improvement of 59% after rehabilitation.

Correlations between Measures for the MRFA and SF-36

Correlations were calculated between the physical functioning and between the affective/mental well-being measures of the MRFA and SF-36. Correlations between scales that are assumed to measure similar constructs were compared to correlations between scales that are assumed to measure different constructs across the MRFA and SF-36 instruments.[3] Table 2 shows that the physical functioning measure (BMC) from the MRFA has a higher correlation with the physical functioning measure (PF) of the SF-36 than with the mental/affective SF-36 measure (MH).

Conversely, the affective well-being measure (Placid) of the MRFA correlates higher with the mental/affective measure (MH) of the SF-36 than with the physical functioning measure (PF) of the SF-36.

Thirdly, intercorrelations between the BMC, Painfree, and Placid measures of the MRFA were examined to verify that each of the measures in the three domains (physical functioning, pain experience, and affective well-being) was measuring a different construct. Table 3 demonstrates that these correlations are relatively low compared to those presented in Table 2 for similar domains across the MRFA and SF-36 measures.

TABLE 2. Correlations between MRFA and SF-36 Rasch Measures at Initial Assessment (N = 94)

	SF-36 Measures		
	Physical		Emotional
MRFA Measures	Physical Functioning		Mental Health
		Physical	
Body Movement and Control	0.83*		0.23
		Emotional	
Placid (Mood and Feelings)	0.11		0.60*

* Significant at 0.01 level

TABLE 3. Correlations among MRFA Measures for Three Domains at Initial Assessment (N = 94)

MRFA Domains	Physical Functioning	Pain Experience	Affective Well-Being
Scale	Body Movement and Control	Painfree	Placid
		Physical functioning	
Body movement and control	—		
		Pain experience	
Painfree	0.24*	—	
		Affective well-being	
Placid	0.13*	0.24*	—

* Non-significant

Therapist Ratings

The criterion validity for the BMC measure of the MRFA was addressed using therapist ratings of improvement in function and change in Rasch measures from before to after rehabilitation. The therapists rated 82% of patients as better, 11% the same, and 7% as worse since beginning rehabilitation. Participants were grouped as better, the same, or worse according to whether their BMC Rasch scores showed improvement, no change, or a decrease from before to after rehabilitation. The Spearman rank order correlation coefficient between change in BMC Rasch measure and rating of improvement was 0.50 ($p < .001$).

SUMMARY AND FUTURE DIRECTIONS

The application of Rasch analysis to the development of the MRFA made possible the construction of linear measures with good clinical precision and acceptable fit characteristics. The results of the reliability and validity studies outlined here support the consistency and usefulness of these measures for persons with musculoskeletal problems. Thus far, development of the MRFA measures has resulted in musculoskeletal, neurologic, and multiple sclerosis forms. Forms for pulmonary, cardiac, and temporomandibular joint problems are currently under development. The next step in examining the validity of the MRFA measures will involve additional studies among persons with various types of problems. These studies, with existing forms and other forms under development, will provide an opportunity to further examine the usefulness and generalizability of the MRFA measures.

The wide variety of problems seen in outpatient rehabilitation settings, as well as the diversity and complexity of living situations, calls for the assessment of many different domains or dimensions of functioning. An example of an area of functioning in the psychosocial domain is the repertoire of ways in which a person copes with environmental stressors. Assessment of improvements in this area of functioning can yield important information relevant to everyday functioning. Among other domains to be assessed with persons living in the community, the role functioning domain is of primary importance. This domain, which includes work, social, and leisure roles, can be considered generic to the variety of problems seen in outpatient settings and essential to improvement of daily living.

Changes in the health care environment have led to a greater emphasis on treatment effectiveness and measurable outcomes. As medical rehabilitation moves increasingly in the direction of community-based treatment, the contribution of Rasch analysis to developing measures that assess single dimensions among many dimensions becomes crucial to outpatient functional assessment and to the measurement of overall quality of daily living.

REFERENCES

1. Baker JG, Granger CV, Fiedler RC: A brief outpatient functional assessment measure: Validity using Rasch measures. Am J Phys Med Rehabil 76:8–13, 1997.
2. Baker JG, Granger CV, Ottenbacher KJ: Validity of a brief outpatient functional assessment measure. Am J Phys Med Rehabil 75:356–363, 1996.
3. Campbell DT, Fiske DW: Convergent and discriminant validation by the mulitrait-multimethod matrix. Psychol Bull 56:81–105, 1959.
4. Derogatis LR, Melisaratos N: The brief symptom inventory: An introductory report. Psychol Med 13:595–605, 1983.
5. Fairbank JC, Couper J, Davies JB, O'Brien JP: The Oswestry low back pain disability questionnaire. Physiotherapy 66:271–273, 1980.
6. Granger CV, Ottenbacker KJ, Baker JG, Sehgal A: Reliability of a brief outpatient functional outcome assessment measure. Am J Phys Med Rehabil 74:469–475, 1995.
7. Granger CV, Seltzer GB, Fishbein CF: The functional assessment. In Granger CV, Seltzer GB, Fishbein CF (eds): Primary Care of the Functionally Disabled: Assessment and Management. New York, Academic Press, 1987.
8. Granger CV, Wright BD: Looking ahead to the use of functional assessment in ambulatory physiatric and primary care: The functional assessment screening questionnaire. Phys Med Rehabil Clin North Am 4:1–11, 1993.
9. Haley SM, McHorney CA, Ware JE: Evaluation of the MOS SF-36 Physical Functioning Scale (PF-10): I. Unidimensionality and reproducibility of the Rasch item scale. J Clin Epidemiol 47:671–684, 1994.
10. Linacre JM, Wright BD: A User's Guide to BIGSTEPS: Rasch Model Computer Program. Chicago, MESA Press, 1992.
11. Melzack R: The short form McGill Pain Questionnaire. Pain 30:191–197, 1987.
12. Tesio L, Granger CV, Fiedler RC: A unidimensional pain/disability measure for low-back pain syndromes. Pain 69:269–278, 1997.
13. Ware JE: SF-36 Health Survey: Manual and Interpretation Guide. Boston, The Health Institute of New England Medical Center, 1993.

JOHN M. LINACRE, PhD

INSTANTANEOUS MEASUREMENT AND DIAGNOSIS

From the MESA Psychometric Laboratory
University of Chicago
Chicago, Illinois

Reprint requests to:
John M. Linacre, PhD
5835 S. Kimbark Ave.
Chicago, IL 60637

BETTER MEASUREMENT

Better measuring instruments are not only more accurate and precise*, they are also more immediate and intuitive. In industrial instrumentation, "better measurements, and more of them, have made it possible to interpret most data without recourse to statistical techniques."[11]

Statistical techniques, particularly as implemented in computer programs, enable the calibration of observation instruments, such as the Functional Independence Measure (FIM), on large samples of patient records, representing many impairment groups and rehabilitation institutions. Collecting and analyzing large patient-record databases is expensive and time-consuming, and although this process yields useful information about the FIM and the patients to which it has been applied,[2] it is far too slow and cumbersome to assist in the treatment of any of the patients whose records are in the database.

Effective use of the FIM requires that data collection, analysis, and interpretation occur almost instantaneously, preferably while the clinician is still with the patient or at least within a day or two. The increasing speed and ubiquity of computers will ultimately permit the development of artificially intelligent systems to support the real-time analysis and interpretation of a patient's ratings on the 18 FIM items. Such interpretation will

* "The term *accuracy* usually denotes in some sense the closeness of the measured values to the true value, taking into consideration both precision and bias. Bias [is] defined as the difference between the limiting mean [of observation] and the true value."[4] Also see, "Use of the Terms *Precision* and *Accuracy* as Applied to the Measurement of a Property of Material" (ASTM Designation, E177-61T, 1961).

be based on the accumulated case histories of millions of patients to whom the FIM will have been administered. Nevertheless, the immediate local clinical experience of practitioners and their personal knowledge of the particular patient will always play a part in FIM interpretation.

Most of the benefits of a sophisticated computer-based system can be realized immediately with the KeyFIM, a simple, paper-and-pencil implementation of the FIM. This form combines into one graphical presentation the essential steps of data collection and measurement construction and a convenient layout for intuitive quality control and diagnostic interpretation.

CALIBRATING THE MEASUREMENT SYSTEM

The FIM consists of 18 items, each rated on a seven-category rating scale with each succeeding category carefully defined to represent an increasing degree of functional independence. It is designed to be administered to patients on admission to and discharge from a rehabilitation institution. Data collected from thousands of applications of the FIM have been subjected to extensive analysis. Linacre et al.[7] report that analysis of FIM data from a measurement perspective by means of the Rasch model discloses that decomposing the 18-item FIM into 13 motor items and the 5 cognitive items produces two bases for measurement clearly superior to the one composite original. For convenience, this paper focuses only on the FIM cognitive items, but the same considerations apply directly to the motor items.

Analysis of the FIM was conducted in the computationally convenient unit of measurement known as the logit (log-odds unit). Other derivations also exist.[6] Although the logit has a clear probabilistic interpretation,[10] its substantive interpretation depends on the use to which the measures are put. FIM measures are used in a rehabilitation setting in which clinicians expect patients to be functioning within a bounded range of the conceptually infinitely wide variable (dimension, construct) of independence. The variable is infinitely wide, because it is always possible to imagine patients even more dependent or independent than any the clinician has already encountered. The bounded range of independence is that for which the rehabilitation setting is designed. Accordingly, it is convenient to define a measurement scale with its 0 point corresponding conceptually to the lowest level of functioning at which a patient might be administered to rehabilitation. Similarly, the 100 point is defined as the highest level of functioning that a patient might achieve and remain in rehabilitation. To maintain the interval-scale measurement characteristics of the logit,[9] this 0–100 scale is a linear transformation of the logit scale. For clarity in substantive use, the new units of measurement are called FIMITs.[5]

TABLE 1. FIM Cognitive Items

	Item Name	FIMIT Calibration
N.	Auditory Comprehension	42
O.	Verbal Expression	40
P.	Social Interaction	46
Q.	Problem Solving	55
R.	Memory	52

Condensed from FIM Guide for the Uniform Data Set for Medical Rehabilitation (Adult FIM). Version 4.0. Buffalo, NY, State University of New York at Buffalo, 1993.

TABLE 2. FIM Rating Scale

No Helper	FIMIT Step Calibration
7. Complete Independence	24
6. Modified Independence	8
Helper	
5. Supervision	1
4. Minimal Assistance	–5
3. Moderate Assistance	–11
2. Maximal Assistance	–17
1. Total Assistance	—

Condensed from FIM Guide for the Uniform Data Set for Medical Rehabilitation (Adult FIM). Version 4.0. Buffalo, NY, State University of New York at Buffalo, 1993.

TABLE 3. Expected FIMIT Measures for Each Level on Each FIM Cognitive Item

	Level						
Item Name	1	2	3	4	5	6	7
N. Auditory Comprehension	8	24	34	41	49	61	82
O. Verbal Expression	5	22	31	39	47	59	80
P. Social Interaction	11	27	37	44	52	64	85
Q. Problem Solving	20	37	46	53	61	73	94
R. Memory	18	34	44	51	59	71	92

Tables of corresponding values of FIM raw scores and FIM measures (in FIMITs) are given in Heinemann et al.[3] along with item calibrations in logits. For the purposes of constructing the KeyFIM, the cognitive score-to-measure conversion table was recomputed by the author based on a random sample of 15,439 relevant patient records from the Uniform Data System (UDS) database using the BIGSTEPS computer program.[8] For the purposes of constructing the KeyFIM, a useful substantive range was obtained when the linear conversion is 12.5 FIMITs per logit. Table 1 contains FIMIT calibrations for the FIM item difficulties for this sample, Table 2 contains FIMIT calibrations for the adjacent category (step) calibrations, and Table 3 contains the expected FIMIT measure corresponding to each possible rating on each FIM item. Since the expected measure for an extreme category is infinite, i.e., out of the operational range of the FIM, a Bayesian adjustment* is made so that, for the extreme categories 1 and 7, the measures corresponding to expected FIM ratings of 1.25 and 6.75 are listed.

* The Bayesian adjustment for extreme scores and ratings employs this line of reasoning: the KeyFIM would not have been administered to the patient if there were no chance that the patient might have been observed in a nonextreme category. Accordingly, the observation in the extreme category was barely enough to qualify as extreme. For extreme scores, this corresponds to an unobservable raw score that is 0.5 raw score points away from the extreme, i.e., a raw score of 35 out of 35 is treated as a score of 34.5, and a raw score of 5 out of 35 is treated as a score of 5.5. For individual ratings, performances in the range of 1.5 to 2.5 would be observed as ratings of level 2. Ratings less than 1.5 would be observed in the extreme levels of 1. Consequently any performance from 1 to 1.5 is observed as 1, and a 1 is treated as an average rating of 1.25 for the purposes of locating the category on the KeyFIM. Similarly, a 7 is treated as a 6.75.

TABLE 4. Conversion Table to Change FIM Raw Scores to FIMIT Measures

FIM Raw Score on 5 Cognitive Items	FIMIT Measure	FIMIT Standard Error
5	0	17
6	8	12
7	17	9
8	22	7
9	25	6
10	28	6
11	30	5
12	32	5
13	34	5
14	36	5
15	38	5
16	40	4
17	41	4
18	43	4
19	44	4
20	46	4
21	47	4
22	49	4
23	51	5
24	52	5
25	54	5
26	56	5
27	58	5
28	61	6
29	63	6
30	67	6
31	70	7
32	75	8
33	81	10
34	91	13
35	100	18

For most IGCs (except 1.1, 2, 12)

Table 4 contains a FIM cognitive raw score to FIMIT measure conversion table. This covers most impairment group codes, except groups 1.1 (left-hemisphere stroke), 2 (brain dysfunction), and 12 (congenital deformity).

CONSTRUCTING THE KEYFIM

The measures and calibrations presented in Tables 1–4 are sufficient to draw the KeyFIM shown in Figure 1. To explain its features and demonstrate its use, the analysis of two patient records is described here.

Figure 2 shows an actual patient record from IGC group 13, "Other Impairments." The KeyFIM has been turned on its side and the FIM levels recorded for each of the five cognitive items (i.e., 3 on item "N. Comprehension"). The FIM ratings total 16. The corresponding levels are circled in the body of the KeyFIM. Data collection is now completed.

Figure 3 depicts the analysis stage. The KeyFIM is rotated and a line drawn through the FIM raw score of 16 in each of three columns. The column "FIM at +1 S.E." indicates a high measure corresponding to one standard error of measurement above the expected measure. The "Linear FIMITs" column indicates that a

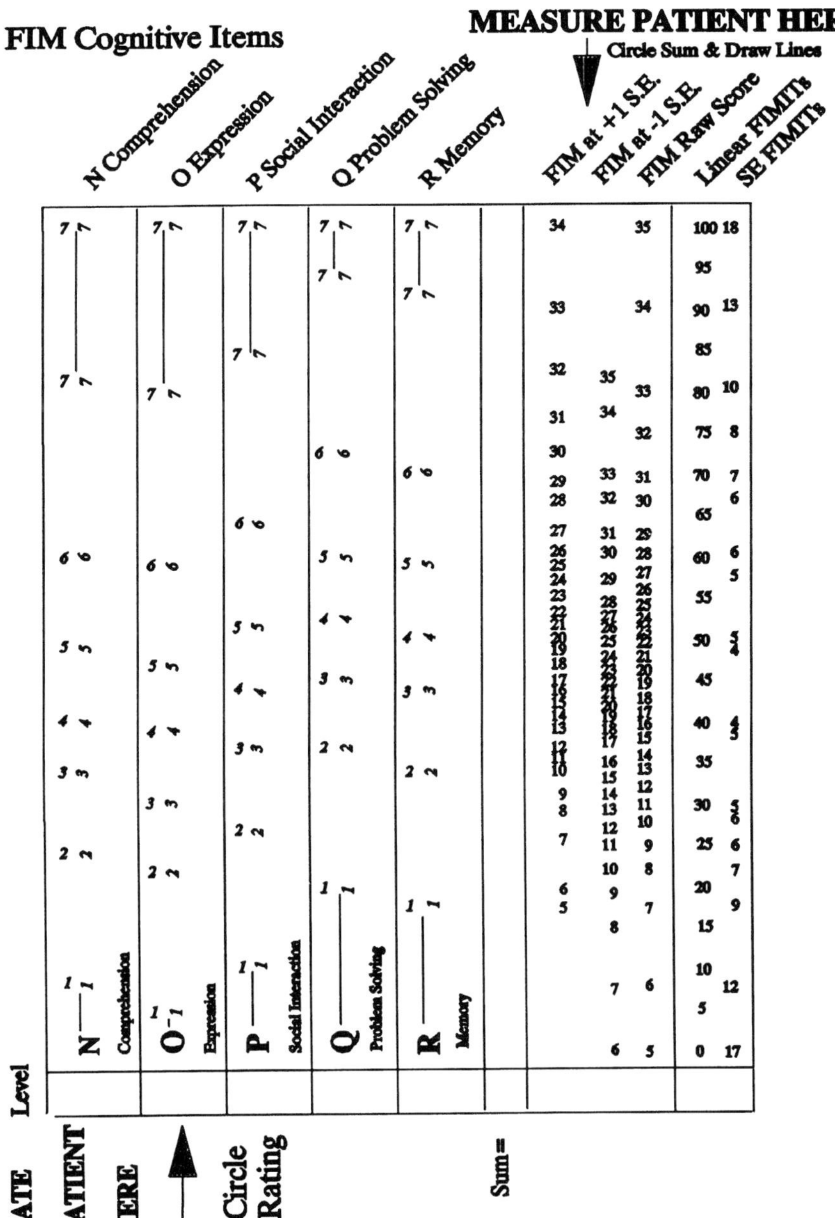

FIGURE 1. KeyFIM data collection and analysis sheet for rating unexpectedness: 1 S.E. ≈ 15 FIMITs.

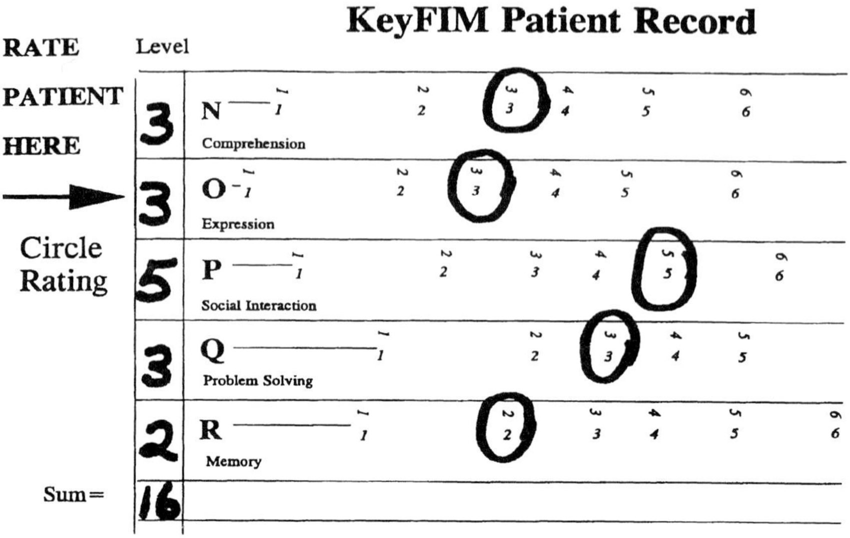

FIGURE 2. KeyFIM data collection.

high measure corresponding to a raw score of 16 is about 45 FIMITs. The column, "FIM at –1 S.E." indicates a low measure one standard error below the expected measure. The "Linear FIMITs" column indicates that this is about 35 FIMITs. The third column, "FIM Raw Score," indicates that the expected measure for a score of 16 is about 40 FIMITs. The right-most column indicates that the standard error measures about ±4 FIMITs, i.e., about the range 35–45. The bottom of the figure states "For Rating Unexpectedness: 1 S.E. ≈ 15 FIMITs." Based on conventional statistical testing, observations located further than 30 FIMITs from the mean line would be suspect, but here the most outlying, 5 on Social Interaction, is only 15 FIMITs away.

In this example there are no observations in extreme categories, but these require special treatment. A rating at an extreme level 1 or 7 corresponds to an infinite range of performance away from the next most extreme category. Accordingly, this is shown by a "__" on the KeyFIM. Thus for 7 on N. Comprehension, the KeyFIM has 7__7. This means that any location along the "__" is a reasonable location for the rating to be marked on the form. In practice, ring around the entire region, as in Figure 4, and choose the point on the line most consistent with the other ratings for measurement and fit analysis purposes.

Instantaneous Measurement and Diagnosis

Since each FIM item provides a locally independent measure of functional independence, FIMs can be used as the basis for an intuitive rather than statistical measurement process. Figure 5 provides an example of another patient record. Here the observation to item "R. Memory" has been deliberately omitted—as though it were not yet recorded, perhaps never to be. Because there is no "complete" raw score, the horizontal lines cannot be drawn directly. Intuitively, it is clear that the patient's typical level of independence is described by the higher

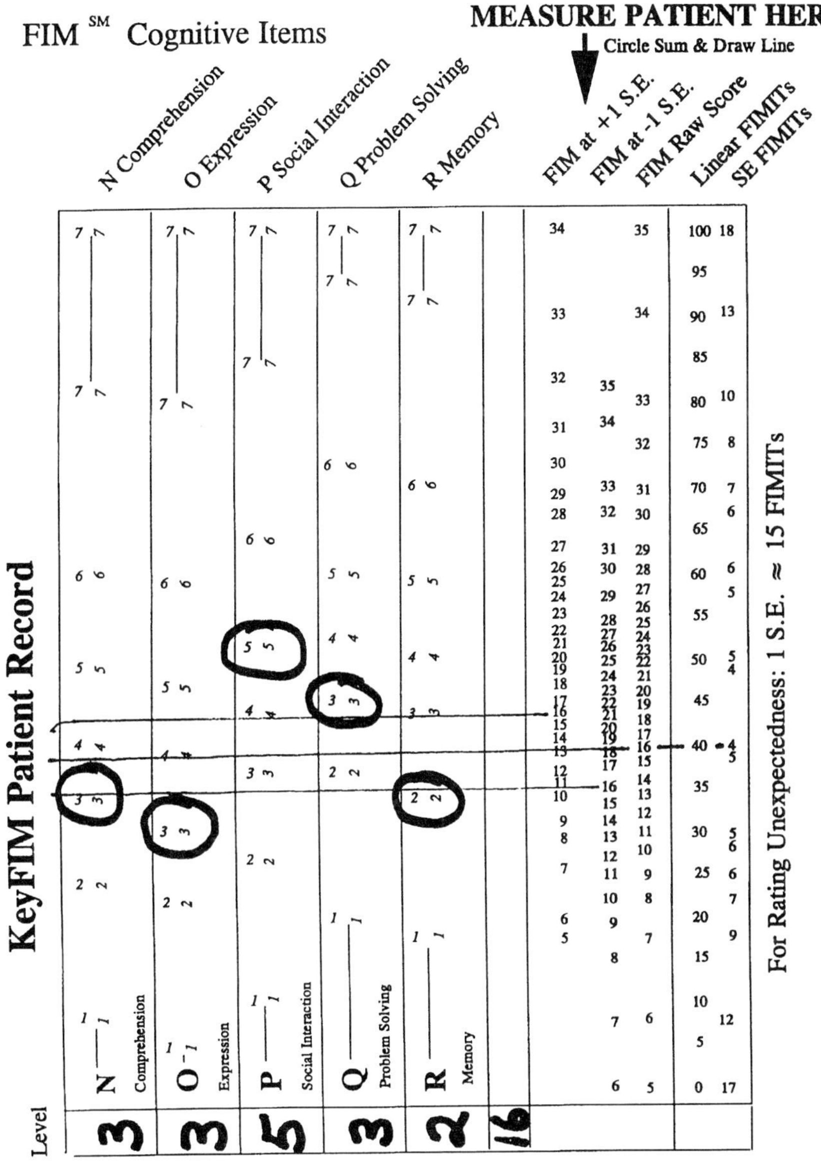

FIGURE 3. KeyFIM measurement and fit diagnosis.

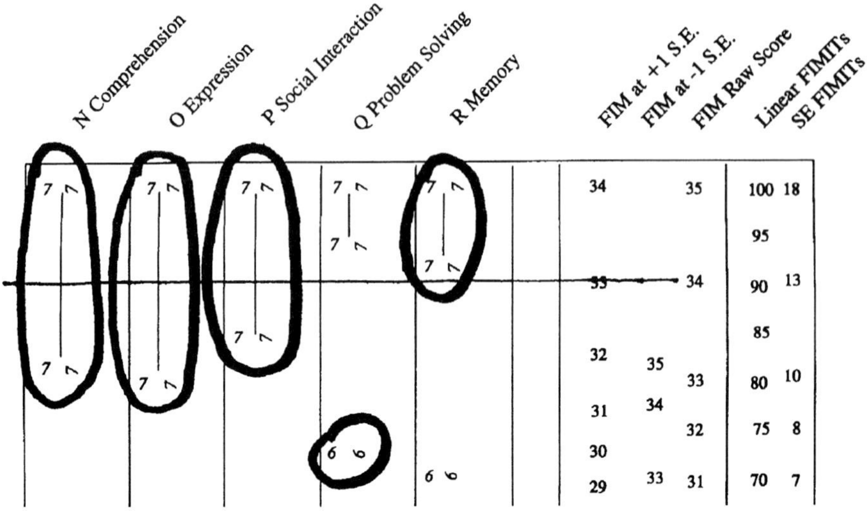

FIGURE 4. Locating extreme ratings on the KeyFIM.

ratings. A line has been drawn by eye through these, yielding a general independence of 58 FIMITs. The S.E. of this measure will be greater than the indicated 5 FIMITs; due to the missing observation and discrepant rating pattern, treating the precision of this measure as ±8 FIMITs would be reasonable. The low rating of 2 on Expression is at 20 FIMITs, about 38 FIMITs below the typical level. Thirty-eight FIMITs is twice the rating S.E. of 15 FIMITs, so that this rating is statistically unexpected. More important for practice, however, is that it is obviously an outlier. For clinical practice, this rating will motivate the patient's immediate therapy.

In this example, measurement and fit diagnosis proceeded successfully and immediately despite incomplete data and the inability to use a "complete" raw score as the basis of analysis. Further, fit analysis and diagnosis could have proceeded successfully even without any formal statistical tests.

CONCLUSION

The KeyFIM is an example of how any rating instrument can be presented as a self-measuring form, supporting intuitive measurement and fit diagnosis. Its format encourages the practitioner to evaluate the ratings as they are being collected, thereby avoiding obvious data entry errors and misunderstandings. With a little experience, the practitioner can perform measurement and fit analysis in the same immediate, effortless, and routine way that useful measurements are obtained from bathroom scales and clinical thermometers. The KeyFIM and instruments like it further blur the artificial distinction between physical and psychological measurement.

REFERENCES

1. FIM Guide for the Uniform Data Set for Medical Rehabilitation (Adult FIM). Version 4.0. Buffalo, NY, State University of New York at Buffalo, 1993.
2. Granger CV, Hamilton BB, Linacre JM, et al: Performance profiles of the Functional Independence Measure. Am J Phys Med Rehabil 72:84–89, 1993.

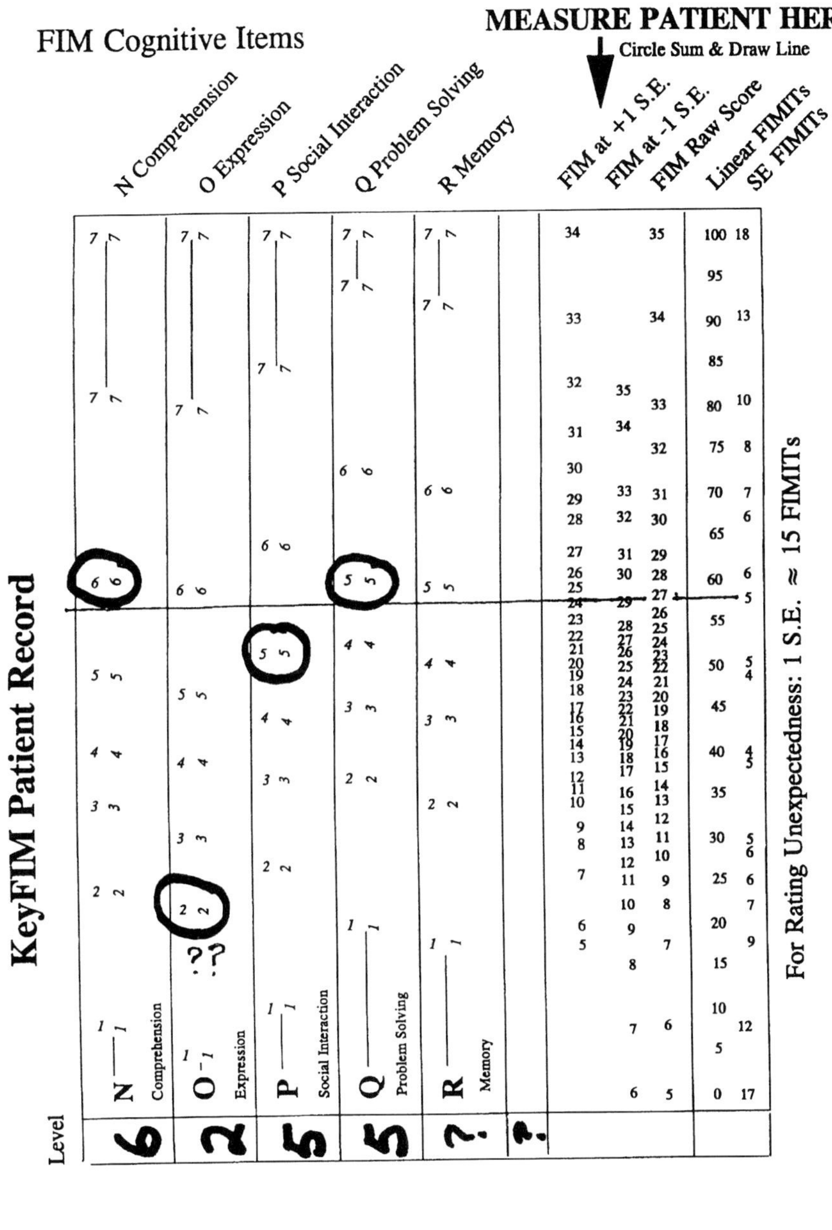

FIGURE 5. KeyFIM intuitive measurement and diagnosis.

3. Heinemann AW, Linacre JM, Wright BD, et al: Measurement characteristics of the Functional Independence Measure. Top Stroke Rehabil 1:1–15, 1994.
4. Ku HH: Statistical concepts in metrology. In Handbook of Industrial Metrology. American Society of Tool and Manufacturing Engineers. New York, Prentice-Hall, 1967, pp 20–50.
5. Linacre JM: KeyFIM—Self-Measuring Score Form. Rasch Measure Trans 9:453–454, 1995.
6. Linacre JM: Why logistic ogive and not autocatalytic curve? Rasch Measure Trans 6:260–261, 1993.
7. Linacre JM, Heinemann AW, Wright BD, et al: The structure and stability of the Functional Independence Measure. Arch Phys Med Rehabil 75:127–132, 1994.
8. Linacre JM, Wright BD: BIGSTEPS Rasch Measurement Computer Program. Chicago, MESA Press, 1991.
9. Stevens SS (ed): Handbook of Experimental Psychology. New York, Wiley, 1951.
10. Wright BD, Stone MH: Best Test Design. Chicago, MESA Press, 1979.
11. Youden WH: Instrumental drift. Science 120:627–631, 1954.

JIN-SHEI LAI, PHD, OTR
CRAIG A. VELOZO, PHD, OTR
JOHN M. LINACRE, PHD

ADJUSTING FOR RATER SEVERITY IN AN UNLINKED FUNCTIONAL INDEPENDENCE MEASURE NATIONAL DATABASE: AN APPLICATION OF THE MANY FACETS RASCH MODEL

From the Department of Occupational Therapy
College of Associated Health Professions
University of Illinois at Chicago (J-SL, CAV)
and
MESA
University of Chicago (JML)
Chicago, Illinois

Reprint requests to:
Jin-Shei Lai, PhD, OTR
Department of Occupational Therapy
College of Associated Health Professions
University of Illinois at Chicago
1919 W. Taylor Avenue
Chicago, IL 60612

Interrater reliability traditionally has been one of the gold standards for determining the quality of measurement instruments in the social sciences. Despite this designation, attempts to improve reliability among raters through the use of standardized grading criteria, administration procedures, and rater training have failed to control the subjectivity of rater assessments.[9,10]

Not only do raters continue to differ in severity, despite extensive efforts at eliminating the differences, rater severities are likely to mask the objective measurement of an individual's ability. The effect is that individuals who are rated by severe raters are likely to achieve scores that are "biased low" while individuals who are rated by lenient raters are likely to achieve scores that are "biased high." Considering the potential effects of rater severity, it is important to determine the influence of raters upon measures. In addition, if this influence is relevant, it would be prudent to adjust measures to account for rater-induced biases.

A number of investigators have demonstrated that the effect of rater severity is not random and that it can have a demonstrable influence on individual scores.[1,2,9,10,12] Furthermore, these researchers have demonstrated the usefulness of item response models to adjust measures for differences in rater severities. Facets, a generalization of the Rasch measurement model, provides a framework for examining performance assessments that include multiple facets, such as rater severity, item difficulty, and ability.[1,7] In contrast to traditional analytic techniques, the "many facets Rasch models" can identify rater biases and remove the bias from the individual's measure.[9]

While measurement models such as facets allow for the detection of and adjustment for rater severity, as with any analysis of rater severity, the one requirement for analysis is some linking of raters. "Linking" refers to having common ratings across raters to allow the calibration of each rater's severity. The requirement of linking provides a unique dilemma for national databases in which the data are generally not linked across raters. Technically, the potential of rater-severity bias has not been identified or corrected in these extensively used data sources due to this problem of unlinked raters. If mechanisms could be designed to link raters in national databases, the influence of rater severity could be identified and measures could be adjusted as needed.

The purpose of this study was to mathematically link unlinked data in a national database of rehabilitation data to account for the effects of rater severity. We applied this linking methodology to a practical application, the adjustment of the functional independence measure (FIM) to control for differences in raters across rehabilitation sites. The FIM, a measure of burden of care, is a widely used indicator of the outcomes of rehabilitation facilities nationally and internationally. Because admission FIM scores are among the most important predictors of critical outcomes such as discharge functional status and length of stay, it is logical to attempt to equate these measures across facilities.[5,6,11] As with other methods of severity adjustment, equating facilities on admission FIM scores would assist in preventing facilities from being penalized for admitting and treating severely impaired patients. The premise of this study was that rater severity may account for differences in admission FIM measures across facilities. Furthermore, through a mathematical linking of this unlinked data and the use of the many facets Rasch model, differences across facilities could be reduced or eliminated.

METHODOLOGY

Sample

The scale analyzed included the 14 motoric items from the FIM scale (eating, grooming, bathing, dressing–upper body, dressing–lower body, toileting, bladder management, bowel management, transfer–bed/chair/wheelchair, transfer–toilet, transfer–tub/shower, walk, wheelchair, and stairs) that have been used as a unidimensional scale.[4] Data for this study were obtained from Formations in Health Care, Inc., in 1995. A total of 1044 patients across different diagnoses were randomly selected from a data set of 11,435 patients. The sample represented 57 facilities and 220 raters.

Data Analysis

Pretest

The initial testing involved using analysis of variance (ANOVA) to examine if patients' average FIM motoric ability measures differed across the 57 facilities. A common assumption is that clinical sites differ in terms of the severity of patients that they admit. To verify this assumption, ANOVA was employed. The basis of all further severity adjustment across facilities was predicated on the finding that the admission FIM motoric measures differ across facilities

RATER SEVERITY ADJUSTMENT

The many facets Rasch analysis program, FACETS,[7] was employed to adjust the possible bias resulting from raters. The basic formula is

$$\log [P_{nijk}/P_{nijk-1}] = B_n - D_i - C_j - F_{ik}$$

where

P_{nijk} = probability of patient n being rated k on domain i by rater j,
P_{nijk-1} = probability of patient n being rated k-1 on domain i by rater j,
B_n = ability of the examinee,
D_i = difficulty of an item,
C_j = severity of a rater,
F_{ik} = difficulty of rating step k relative to step k-1.

The assumption is that each observed rating is the probabilistic result of four interacting components: the ability of an examinee, the difficulty of an item, the severity of a rater, and the structure of the rating scale.[8] An underlying assumption is that the rating derived from behavioral observations always contains some rater subjectivities. The goal of measurement is to reduce the possible subjectivity across raters as much as possible.[1–3,9,10,12]

LINKING RATERS IN AN UNLINKED DATABASE

Due to the nature of the FIM database, since raters evaluated patients in their own facility, there was no linkage across raters and facilities. Therefore, a mechanism to link raters was employed based upon the concept of variance. This methodology is not intended to totally eliminate rater biases but, instead, to decrease the bias resulting from raters as much as possible. A three-step procedure was used (Table 1).

Step 1 involved analyzing only subject and item facets. In this step, the rating each subject obtained was the log linear combination of the item, the subject, and random error. An underlying assumption in this step is that raters were identical; therefore, when considering an observed rating, rater severity was not taken into account. Subject measures obtained from step 1 represented the combination of the subject and rater effects, since the subject and the rater are mutually influenced to some degree. Therefore, in step 1, the variance of the subject is maximized, since the rater effects were included in subject measures.

Step 2 involved analyzing another combination of facets, rater, and item. In this step, the rating each subject obtained was the log linear combination of the rater,

TABLE 1. A Three-Step Process to Decrease Bias among Raters

Procedure	Rationale	NB
Step 1	Rating = Subject + Item + Error	∵ Subject = Subject Ability + Rater Effects
		∴ Subject variance is maximized
Step 2	Rating = Rater + Item + Error	∵ Rater = Rater Severity + Subject Effects ∴
		∴ Rater variance is maximized
Step 3	Rating = Subject + Rater + Item + Error	∵ Subject Ability
		∴ Subject variance is minimized

Notes: Rater was anchored with the value of rater measures at Step 2 × Item SD1/SD2.
Item was stable across different steps and was anchored with the value obtained from Step 1.

Although rater severity is known to contribute to the biasing of measures, other factors also are likely to contribute to differences across facilities in admission FIM measures. While the present study used the many facets Rasch model to adjust scores for rater severity, this methodology also can be used to adjust measures for factors such as age, diagnosis, and comorbidities. It would be interesting to determine if facilities could be equated if admission FIM measures were corrected for factors other than rater severity.

In contrast to traditional statistical techniques, the many facets Rasch model adjusts not just grouped scores but individual measures. Therefore, a subject's true measure of ability can be more closely approximated. The advantage of adjusting individual measures is that we are less likely to misinterpret an individual's performance that may have been biased by factors that mask the true ability we are trying to measure.

The major challenge faced in this study was to adjust for rater severity using data that was not linked across raters. Resolving this problem has practical significance, since most existing databases consist of unlinked data. To meet this challenge, data were linked mathematically. The underlying assumption was that all raters are linked, since they all use the same items. Through a logical series of separate analyses and anchoring the final analysis on the basis of previous analyses, the final measures were adjusted for rater severity. This methodology provides a correction mechanism for unlinked databases that was not previously available.

This study suggests that rater severities influence FIM measures and can be adjusted using the many facets Rasch model. Furthermore, this study presents a logical mechanism to correct for rater severity in unlinked data. Clearly, this is not the ideal mechanism for correcting data for rater severity; however, because the data in national databases are unlinked, the choice of correction techniques is limited. The empirical test of this methodology is to compare the results of mathematical linking to traditional linking on the same linked data. Only if the results are similar can mathematical linking be validated as an approach for rater severity adjustment in unlinked data.

REFERENCES

1. Englehard G: Examining rater errors in the assessment of written composition with a many-faceted Rasch model. J Educ Measure 31:93–112, 1994.
2. Fisher AG: The assessment of IADL motor skills: An application of many-faceted Rasch analysis. Am J Occup Ther 47:319–329, 1993.
3. Forsyth K, Lai J, Kielhofner G: The assessment of communication and interaction skills (ACIS). Am J Occup Ther (in press).
4. Granger CV, Hamilton BB, Linacre JM, et al: Performance profiles of the functional independence measure. Am J Phys Med Rehabil 72:84–89, 1993.
5. Heinemann AW, Linacre JM, Wright BD, et al: Prediction of rehabilitation outcomes with disability measures. Arch Phys Med Rehabil 75:133–143, 1994.
6. Hosek S, Kane R, Carney M, et al: Charges and Outcomes for Rehabilitative Care: Implications for the Prospective Payment System. Santa Monica, CA, Rand, 1986.
7. Linacre JM: FACETS Computer Program for Many-Faceted Rasch Measurement. Chicago, MESA Press, 1994.
8. Linacre JM: Many-Faceted Rasch Measurement. Chicago, MESA Press, 1994.
9. Lunz ME, Stahl JA: The effect of rater severity on person ability measure: A Rasch model analysis. Am J Occup Ther 47:311–317, 1993.
10. Lunz ME, Wright B, Linacre M: Measuring the impact of judge severity on examination scores. Appl Measure Educ 3:331–345, 1990.
11. National Association of Rehabilitation Facilities: A prospective payment system for inpatient medical rehabilitation services [position paper and study]; final report. Washington, DC, NARF, 1985.
12. Wilson M, Wang W: Complex composites: Issues that arise in combining different modes of assessment. Appl Psychol Measure 19:51–71, 1995.

RICHARD M. SMITH, PhD

THE RELATIONSHIP BETWEEN GOALS AND FUNCTIONAL STATUS IN THE PATIENT EVALUATION AND CONFERENCE SYSTEM

From the Rehabilitation Foundation Inc.
Marianjoy Rehabilitation Hospital and Clinics
Wheaton, Illinois

Reprint requests to:
Richard M. Smith, PhD
Rehabilitation Foundation Inc.
26W171 Roosevelt Road
Wheaton, IL 60187

Much of the research in outcome measurement has been devoted to the establishment of interval scales to facilitate the analysis and interpretations of rehabilitation outcomes. There are several examples of the successful application of Rasch measurement models to outcome data, including the Patient Evaluation and Conference System (PECS),[3] the Functional Independence Measure (FIM),[4] and LORS.[12] These systems are based primarily on the evaluation of the patient's status at various points in the rehabilitation process. Status is usually measured at admission and discharge but may be evaluated more frequently. Functional gains are often calculated from these evaluations as the difference between admission and discharge scores. As Wright reports in the opening chapter, for these gains to have meaning, the items must be measured on an interval scale so that the differences are appropriate for the usual types of parametric statistical analysis. One way functional gains can be used in program evaluation is to compare them to historical data collected at the local, regional, or national level. For instance, how do this quarter's gains in toilet transfers compare with the average gains in the program for the last 2 years? There are two major drawbacks to using this type of comparison to evaluate programs. The first drawback is that the standard errors for the item level observations are not known, even when an item is measured on an interval scale (which is rarely the case). One can never be sure that progressing from a 3 to a 4 represents a real change or if the two values are within standard errors of each other and represent only measurement error. The second drawback is that comparisons to historical standards must be done on an item-by-item basis. The FIM allows 18 possible comparisons between functional gains and historical averages. The interpretation of this pattern for a particular diagnostic group is often difficult to summarize and is even more difficult when combined across diagnostic groups that have different patterns of gains.

Wright points out in the opening chapter that the use of Rasch measurement models in the analysis of these types of data can be helpful in several ways. First, when the data fit the model, the resulting measures of status must be on an interval scale, and research has shown that most outcome scales fit one of the family of Rasch measurement models. Second, the model allows the summarization of items that measure a common theme into unidimensional measures that have known standard errors. The summarization of items into linear unidimensional scales greatly facilitates interpretation. In the case of the FIM, the 18 ordinal observations are reduced into two unidimensional interval measures with known standard errors.[4] Thus, the comparison of current measures with historical results is made easier because the comparison involves only the motor skills and cognition scales rather than 18 separate items.

There is a drawback to using only historical comparisons in program evaluation: this approach makes certain assumptions about the initial severity of the patient's condition as well as the number and severity of comorbidities. Other assumptions about the diagnostic mix may be necessary if the gains are compared at a facility level across diagnostic groups. The use of historical comparisons only also overlooks an important source of information: clinical judgment of potential rehabilitation goals. Clinical judgment can be incorporated into the evaluation process through the use of goals for the rehabilitation stay that are set at admission to the program. If goals are used in program evaluation, the effects of initial severity, comorbidities, and diagnostic mix are controlled by the application of clinical judgment. For example, a person with a severe comorbidity such as a cardiac problem might be expected to make smaller motor skills gains in a stroke program than a patient without the cardiac problem.

The same items used to measure functional status often are used to establish short-term (discharge) and long-term (postdischarge) goals for the patient. However, the use of these item sets to measure goals is based on two assumptions: (1) the use of the status items to set goals results in a unidimensional variable, i.e., the data must fit the psychometric model chosen; and (2) the status and goal scales define the same underlying variable. If a comparison between the goals set at admission and the functional status at discharge is to be used as an effective measure of the rehabilitation process, the two measures must be on the same metric. Otherwise, differences that might be used in summary statistics will have no directly interpretable meaning. Few studies have verified the assumptions of unidimensional scales or common metrics for status and goal scales.

This chapter reports on the investigation of the interval scale properties of measures of discharge goals based on the items from the Patient Evaluation and Conference System functional status scales, and it establishes that the measures from the goal scales can be statistically combined with measures of functional assessment to produce estimates of goal attainment in the rehabilitation process. Finally, goal and status measures are used to describe rehabilitation progress in stroke and musculoskeletal rehabilitation programs.

PECS is a comprehensive patient tracking system designed to assess the functional status of persons involved in physical rehabilitation. It is an interdisciplinary evaluation tool that draws on the major clinical areas in the rehabilitation team: physician, nurse, occupational therapist, physical therapist, speech language pathologist, psychologist, neuropsychologist, social worker, therapeutic recreation specialist, and vocational counselor. The current PECS system contains more than 140 items organized into six unidimensional LifeScales: rehabilitation medicine, applied self-care, motor skills, community reintegration, cognition and communication, and pain.

METHODS

In many Rasch-based studies, the similarity of the underlying variable in different applications is assessed by comparing calibrations from different diagnostic groups, such as stroke and brain-injured patients.[2] The multiple calibration technique produces estimates of the item difficulty as well as the asymptotic standard errors for the item measures. Since the same items are used in both calibrations, the arbitrary zero of the logit scale is set to the same point, the mean item difficulty. The differences between the item measures for the two calibrations can be identified using the t-test approach.[16] It is also possible to make a bivariate plot of the item measures (difficulties) and construct two standard error bands around the unit slope line, which is the expected pattern for the plots.[16] This allows one to distinguish between items whose differences are likely due to measurement error and those likely to be real differences between the two groups or applications of interest. Both of these techniques work well when only two groups are being compared, but for three or more groups only pairwise comparisons are possible and family-wide Type I error rates might become an issue. One way around this problem is to use the item between-group fit statistic that provides a single test for any number of groups.[8] This statistic is based on a single calibration of the data.

The BIGSTEPS program[14] was used to calibrate the various scales (motor skills, applied self-care and cognition/communication) for both status and goals. BIGSTEPS provides estimates of the item difficulties, asymptotic standard errors, and a variety of fit statistics that can be used in the evaluation of the fit of the data to the model. Person and item separation reliabilities, the ratio of total variance to true variance, are also reported.[15]

DATA

This study uses the separate calibration technique to establish the suitability of the PECS LifeScales to measure functional status and short-term and long-term goals. The study is based on the admission and discharge status evaluations of all patients discharged from a free-standing rehabilitation hospital in 1995. Short-term goals—the discharge goals—were set at admission. The long-term goals—postdischarge goals—were set at discharge. Status and goals were recorded on the same evaluation form by the clinician.

More than 4300 evaluations were included in the analysis, but the number varied across the LifeScales. For instance, only about 2100 patients were evaluated on the cognition/communication items. The data included patients from three levels of care: inpatient, subacute, and day hospital. The rehabilitation goals, determined at admission, and the 1-year goals, determined at discharge, were included in the study. The results for motor skills, cognition/communication, and applied self-care PECS LifeScales are presented in this chapter.

Discipline: PHY (usually completed by Physical Therapist)

PHY1 Transfers
Moving to and from wheelchair to mat table and bed from both directions. Set up for transfer and management of wheelchair parts necessary for safe transfer are included.

0 Not assessed.
1 Maximal assistance: patient attempts to participate or provide some physical assistance in carrying out the activity, but requires significant physical and verbal assistance to complete the activity. Patient is able to assist with up to 25% of the activity.
2 Moderate assistance: patient attempts to participate or provide some physical assistance in carrying out the activity, but requires physical and verbal assistance to complete the activity. Patient is able to assist with 25% - 75% of the activity.
3 Minimal assistance: patient is able to participate fully in the activity, but requires intermittent physical assistance and/or contact guard. Patient is able to assist with 75% or more of the activity.
4 Standby assistance: patient performs the activity without physical/hands on assist. May require verbal cuing, prior demonstration or supervision to complete the activity safely.
5 Limited independent: patient is independent in the activity but requires an assistive device or environmental modification.
6 Functional independent: patient is independent in the activity but demonstrates an altered quality of movement or requires an unreasonable amount of time.
7 Within normal limits: patient is independent in the activity with reaction time and quality of movement appropriate for age.

FIGURE 1. Sample motor skills item from the PECS LifeScales.

The motor skills scale contains 20 items, the cognition/communication scale contains 12 items, and the applied self-care scale contains 8 items. Evaluations for each item were made on a 1–7 point ordinal scale, running from "maximum dependence" (1) to "within normal limits" (7). The ordinal observations were converted into an interval scale using the Rasch partial credit model. The data for each scale were calibrated separately to produce a pair of items difficulties—status and goal—for each of the LifeScales. A sample item from the motor skills scale is shown in Figure 1.

RESULTS

The outcome scales for the goal assessments discussed in this chapter, motor skills, applied self-care, and cognition/communication, were part of a larger study.[11] The use of the three scales to assess goals had similar psychometric properties to the use of the corresponding scales for functional status assessment. The results of the Rasch calibrations of the status and goal assessments are presented in Table 1. Two questions needed to be answered with these data: "Are the items measuring anything?" and "Are the scales unidimensional?" The person and item separation reliabilities give

TABLE 1. Calibration Statistics

Scale	Statistic	Status	Goal
Applied Self-Care	Person Separation Reliability	0.95	0.96
	Item Separation Reliability	0.95	0.96
	OUTFIT MNSQ > 1.25	1/8	1/8
Motor Skills	Person Separation Reliability	0.97	0.97
	Item Separation Reliability	0.96	1.00
	OUTFIT MNSQ > 1.25	4/20	4/20
Cognition/Communication	Person Separation Reliability	0.91	0.90
	Item Separation Reliability	0.92	0.92
	OUTFIT MNSQ > 1.25	2/12	4/12

a good indication of whether the scales measure anything. For the cognition/communication scale, the person and item separation index—the ratio of the true variance to the observed variance—is above 0.90, and it is above 0.95 for the applied self-care and motor skills scales. The person separation reliability is similar to coefficient alpha, often reported in true-score model analyses. The item separation reliability has no complementary statistic in the true-score model. At 0.90 and higher, it is safe to conclude that these scales measure what they are measuring very reliably; there is a small amount of error variance relative to the true variance among the items and the persons. The fact that there are asymptotic standard errors for the estimates of the person and item measures makes it possible to estimate the true variance used in these separation reliabilities. The person and item separation reliabilities for the status and goal calibrations are within 0.01 for the three LifeScales, suggesting that they are equally reliable under both uses.

The extent to which the data fit the model can best be evaluated by the item mean square fit statistic. In most cases, a value of 1.25 can be used to detect misfit. Kilgore et al. use this value in their initial analyses of the PECS LifeScales.[3] At this level the mean squares have a Type I error rate of about 0.03–0.04.[9,10] Only one of the eight applied self-care items and four of the 20 motor skills items have a value greater than 1.25. This is three to four times the Type I error rate, but it indicates that most of the items fit the model. These calibrations were based on a mixture of diagnostic programs, which can lead to slightly different definitions of the motor skills scale.[2] The mixture of diagnostic groups often can cause this misfit. Two of the 12 cognition/communication items misfit on the status calibration, and four of the 12 items misfit on the goal calibration. The frequency of the misfit on the goal calibration is of concern as is the difference in frequency of misfit between the status and goal calibrations. There does not appear to be any systematic reason for this difference, but cognition/communication is the least well defined of the LifeScales. Since the data fit the Rasch partial credit model, the scales also can be said to be unidimensional.[7,13]

Once it has been demonstrated that the scales are unidimensional and are reliable—meaning that they separate the items and persons along a common variable, the only remaining question is whether the status and goal scales for the three LifeScales define the same variable. The separate calibration t-test was used to compare the item difficulties for the status and goal calibrations for the three LifeScales. Given the large sample sizes, the tests are very sensitive; standard errors of estimation for the item measures are extremely small. The bivariate plots of the two calibrations for the three LifeScales are shown in Figures 2–4. The results suggest that the definition of the variable is the same for both status and goals. The applied self-care scale in Figure 2 shows a similar pattern of item difficulty with the exception of one item, interdisciplinary activity. Relative to the rest of the items, this item is more likely to receive a high score in the setting of goals than in the status evaluation. The interdisciplinary activity item moves about four places in item difficulty order when goal and status evaluations are compared. This item requires that the nursing staff assess the patient's ability to perform four activities from any discipline other than applied self-care.

Figure 3 shows a similar pattern for the motor skills items. In this comparison, three of the 20 items should be noted. Endurance, the most difficult item in the status calibration, is more likely to receive higher scores in setting goals. Two other items, car transfers and environmental barriers, are more likely to receive higher scores in the status evaluation than in setting goals. The remainder of the items have similar difficulties across the two settings.

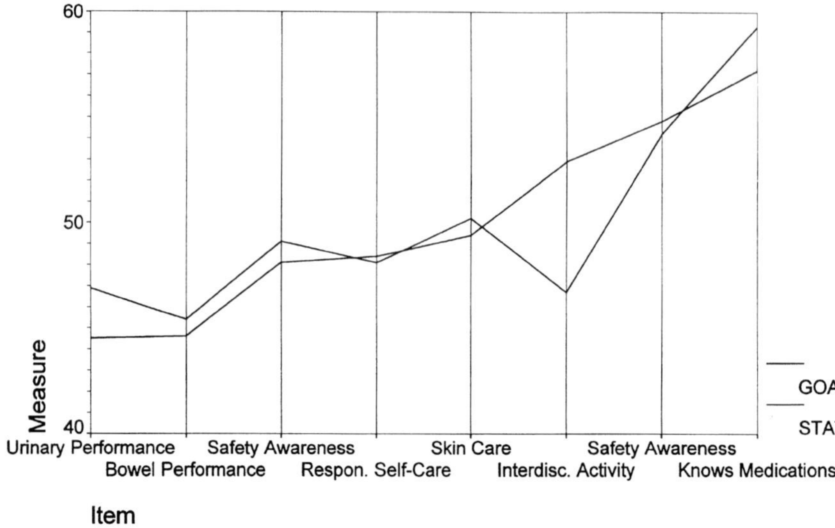

FIGURE 2. Applied self-care items: goal vs. status item measures.

The plot in Figure 4 shows a slightly different pattern for the cognition/communication items. Although there is the same general trend in difficulty across the items, more items have differences between the status and goal difficulty calibrations. One item, comprehending speech, receives lower ratings on goals relative to the rest of the items. Four items receive lower ratings on the status evaluation: produce language, attention concentration impairment, verbal language processing impairment, and basic intellectual skills impairment.

Another method of assessing the extent to which the status and goal evaluations were measuring the same variable is to calculate the correlation between the

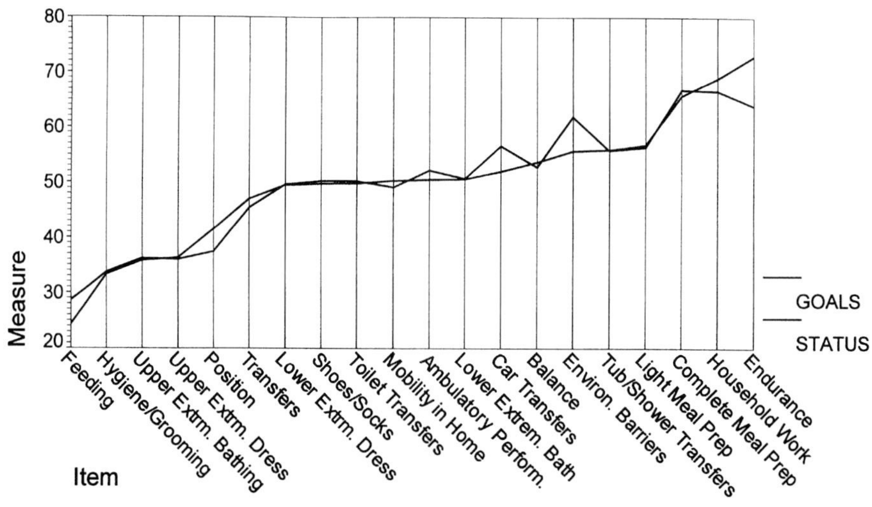

FIGURE 3. Motor skills items: goal vs. status item measures.

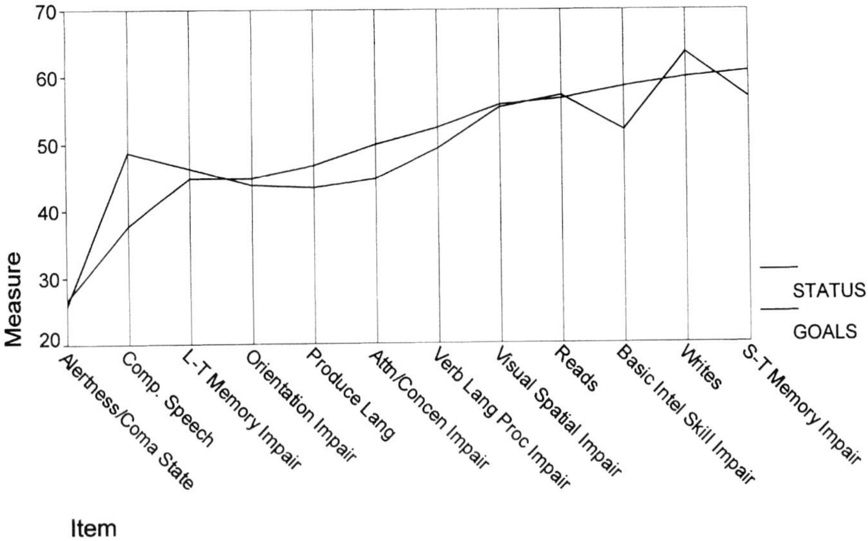

FIGURE 4. Cognition/communication items: goal vs. status item measures.

two sets of item difficulties. The correlation between the motor skills status and goal item difficulties was 0.96, the correlation for the cognition/communication items was 0.89, and the correlation for the applied self-care items was 0.83. The latter is somewhat lower due to the restriction in range of the item difficulties for that scale versus the other two scales. These correlations are not corrected for the presence of measurement error in the estimation of the item difficulties; if they were corrected, they would increase. The values also suggest that the ordering of the item difficulties was similar enough for the scales to be considered as measuring the same variable. This satisfies the assumption that the status and goal scales were measuring the same variable and allows the comparison of rehabilitation goals and discharge status as a means of evaluating the effectiveness of the rehabilitation process.

Once it has been established that the goal and status uses of the LifeScale items are measuring the same underlying variable, it is possible to form differences between the person measures on the goal-setting and status evaluation that can be directly interpreted. Of primary interest is the comparison between the goals of rehabilitation set on admission and the status on discharge. This difference can be used in program evaluation to determine the extent to which a program is meeting the rehabilitation goals. The second part of the study demonstrates that use.

Analysis of Stroke and Musculoskeletal Programs

Included in the second part of the study were 805 persons discharged as "rehab complete" in either the stroke or musculoskeletal programs from a free-standing rehabilitation hospital in 1995. The analysis of the effectiveness of the rehabilitation programs compared initial goals, completed within 1 week of admission, with discharge status on four PECS LifeScales: motor skills (20 items), applied self-care (8 items), cognition/communication (12 items), and community reintegration (13 items). The difference between initial goals and discharge status was calculated as a

TABLE 2. Program Evaluation Results

Scale	Statistics	Stroke Program	Musculoskeletal Program
Applied Self-Care	Initial Status	11	21
	Discharge Status	57	68
	Initial Goals	51	65
Motor Skills	Initial Status	15	32
	Discharge Status	46	56
	Initial Goals	40	54
Cognition/Communication	Initial Status	54	63
	Discharge Status	68	77
	Initial Goals	63	74
Community Reintegration	Initial Status	41	48
	Discharge Status	57	63
	Initial Goals	54	59

means of evaluating the effectiveness of the rehabilitation programs. The average initial status, discharge status, and initial rehabilitation goals for the four LifeScales and the two programs are shown in Table 2. For the stroke and musculoskeletal programs, the discharge status exceeded discharge goals on all four of the LifeScales: stroke—motor skills = +5.33, cognitive/communication = +5.29, community reintegration = +3.11, applied self-care = +6.71; musculoskeletal—motor skills = +1.92, cognitive/communication = +3.77, community reintegration = +3.87, applied self-care = +3.22. Thus, the comparison of the discharge status and the rehabilitation goals provides a picture of the extent to which the rehabilitation goals are being met. This comparison also can be made on an individual basis, reporting the proportion of persons who exceeded the rehabilitation goals on discharge. The chance always exists that there might be a systematic lowering of goals to make a program "look better," but in most cases it seems prudent to trust that the members of the rehabilitation team are using their best clinical judgment to set the goals.

Another area of interest in rehabilitation is the prediction of discharge status on admission. With various proposals for severity-based reimbursement plans being discussed, this topic has engendered renewed interest. Given this background, the correlations of initial status and initial goals, both of which were set on admission, with discharge status were calculated. For the musculoskeletal program, initial goals were a better predictor of discharge status than initial status on all of the LifeScales except community reintegration. For the stroke program, initial goals were a better predictor of discharge status on the applied self-care and motor skills LifeScales. This suggests that initial goals might be useful information to be considered in a severity-based reimbursement system.

DISCUSSION

LifeScale maps discussed by Wright in the opening chapter are the direct result of the Rasch calibration process and are constructed directly from the BIGSTEPS output. These maps can be modified to provide a convenient data collection form for clinicians. The forms provide an item-by-item summary of initial and discharge status and goals, as well as the summary LifeScale scores. The collection of this type of information on a map can highlight areas of progress that are higher or lower than expected. The motor skills LifeScales map for the musculoskeletal and stroke programs used in the previous analysis are shown in Figures 5 and 6.

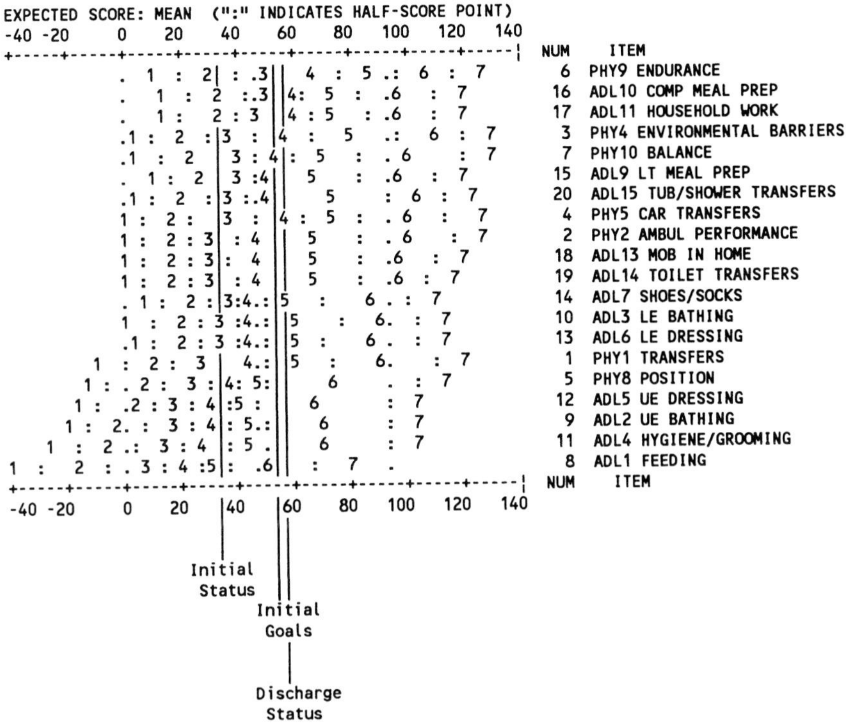

FIGURE 5. Motor skills PECS map, musculoskeletal program.

These maps incorporate normative information such as average initial status, average initial goals, and average discharge status for each of the programs. It is also possible to provide percentile information for admission or discharge status across the bottom of the scale so that the clinician can get an immediate impression of the status of the current patient relative to the historical distribution of initial severity for that program. In some instances the use of hospital-wide data might replace the program-specific data. The maps also are useful in showing the transitions across levels of care. Wright's chapter provides further details on how the maps can be used for controlling the quality of the individual item assessments.

CONCLUSION

The use of goal attainment to measure the effectiveness of treatment programs has been greatly limited by the ordinal nature of most outcome scales. The ordinal nature and the multidimensionality of the scales often make summary scores less than optimal for the calculation of goal attainment. The usual response to the multidimensionality problem is to consider each item on the scale a separate entity for comparison of goals of therapy and outcomes. This strategy has several problems. First, the standard errors associated with the scores are unknown, making it difficult to separate chance differences from real differences. Second, the relatively large number of comparisons—one for each item—make summarization of the overall treatment effectiveness difficult. Third, there is little evidence to support the notion that evaluation goals and status with the same items really measure the same variable.

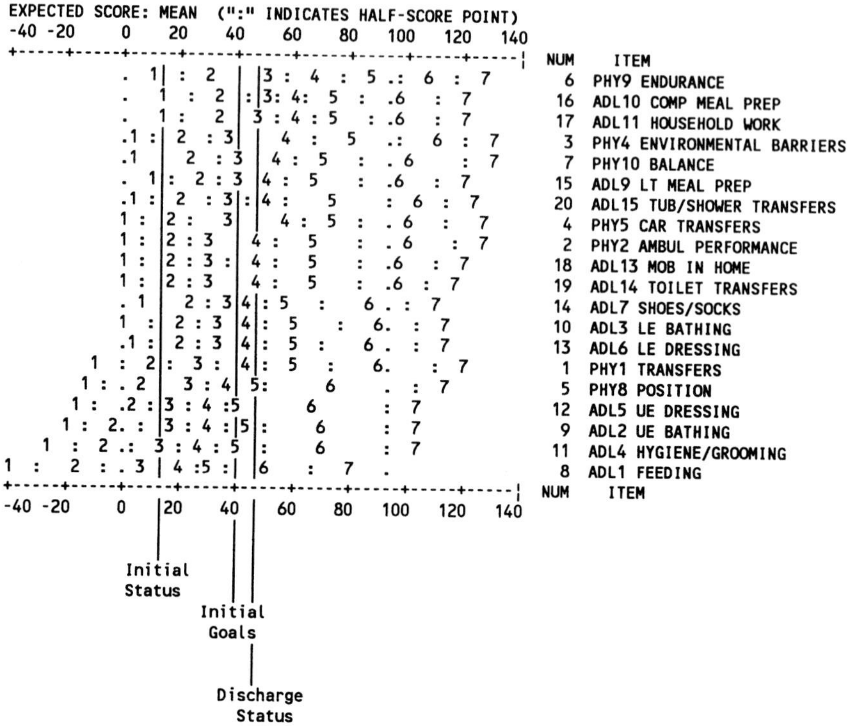

FIGURE 6. Motor skills PECS map, stroke program.

With the increasing use of Rasch models in outcome measurement, many of these methodologic issues can be solved. Using scales that provide interval measures of initial and discharge status and admission and discharge goals provides a summary measure of status and goals that can be analyzed with parametric statistics. It also provides a method of assessing the similarity of the variables assessed for goals and status.

REFERENCES

1. Harvey RP, Silverstein B, Kilgore KM, et al: Applying psychometric criteria to functional assessment in medical rehabilitation: III. Construct validity and predicting level of care. Arch Phys Med Rehabil 73:887–892, 1992.
2. Kilgore KM, Fisher WP, Harvey RF, Silverstein B: Diagnostic-based differences in Rasch calibrations of functional assessment scales. Arch Phys Med Rehabil 74:1254, 1993.
3. Kilgore KM, Fisher WP, Silverstein B, et al: Application of Rasch analysis to the Patient Evaluation and Conference System. Phys Med Rehabil Clin North Am 4:493–515, 1993.
4. Linacre JM, Heinemann AW, Wright BD, et al: The structure and stability of the Functional Independence Measure. Arch Phys Med Rehabil 74:566–573, 1994.
5. Silverstein B, Kilgore KM, Fisher WP, et al: Applying psychometric criteria to functional assessment: I. Exploring unidimensionality. Arch Phys Med Rehabil 72:631–637, 1991.
6. Silverstein B, Kilgore KM, Fisher WP, et al: Applying psychometric criteria to functional assessment in medical rehabilitation: II. Defining interval measures. Arch Phys Med Rehabil 73:507–518, 1992.
7. Smith RM: A comparison of methods for determining dimensionality in Rasch measurement. Structural Equation Modeling 3:25–40, 1996.
8. Smith RM: Applications of Rasch Measurement. Chicago, MESA Press, 1992.

9. Smith RM: IPARM: Item and Person Analysis with the Rasch Model. Chicago, MESA Press, 1991.
10. Smith RM: The distributional properties of Rasch standardized residuals. Educ Psychol Measure 48:657–667, 1988.
11. Smith RM, Wright RE, Harvey RF: Developing linear scales to measure goals of rehabilitation. Arch Phys Med Rehabil 77:969–970, 1996.
12. Velozo CA, Magalhaes LC, Pan A, Leiter P: Functional scale discrimination at admission and discharge: Rasch analysis of the level of rehabilitation Scale III. Arch Phys Med Rehabil 76:705–712, 1995.
13. Wright BD: Comparing Rasch measurement and factor analysis. Structural Equation Modeling 3:1–24, 1996.
14. Wright BD, Linacre JM: BIGSTEPS, A Rasch Model Computer Program. Chicago, MESA Press, 1996.
15. Wright BD, Masters GN: Rating Scale Analysis. Chicago, MESA Press, 1982.
16. Wright BD, Stone MH: Best Test Design. Chicago, MESA Press, 1979.

NORBERT GOLDFIELD, MD, RICHARD F. AVERILL, MS
THELMA GRANT, RRA, YVETTE WANG, MS
DENNIS GRAZIANO, BBA, HERBERT FILLMORE, MA
WILLIAM P. FISHER, JR, PHD

IMPROVING THE PREDICTION OF REHABILITATION OUTPATIENT HEALTH SERVICES USING PATIENT CHARACTERISTICS:

Results of a Six-Month Prospective Study

From 3M Health Information Systems
Wallingford, Connecticut (NG, RFA, TG, YW)
and
New York State Department of Health
New York, New York (DG, HF)
and
Louisiana State University School of Public Health
New Orleans, Louisiana (WF)

Reprint requests to:
Norbert Goldfield, MD
3M Health Information Systems
72 Laurel Park
North Hampton, MA 01060

This chapter was prepared with the support of the Health Care Financing Administration, Office of Research and Demonstrations, under cooperative agreement 17-C-90057/5-01 to 3M Health Information Systems. The opinions expressed are solely those of the authors and do not necessarily represent those of the Health Care Financing Administration.

This study examines whether additional data elements not currently collected on the standard claim form increases the ability of ambulatory patient groups (APGs) to predict resource consumption. This is important to pursue because certain medical services, on the basis of claim form data, have been historically difficult to understand from a resource consumption perspective.

APGs were developed pursuant to a grant from the Health Care Financing Administration as a classification system for ambulatory services. The APGs can be used as the basic unit of payment in a prospective payment system for outpatient services. The initial APG research was completed in December 1990 and resulted in a classification system (APG 1.0) consisting of 298 patient groups covering all outpatient services provided in hospital outpatient departments. The most recent APG research resulted in a second version of the APGs (APG 2.0), consisting of 290 groups, some of which were changed from the first version. Both versions of the APGs use only information present on the existing claim form.

Data not currently collected on the claim form may be useful for clinical areas that historically have not been well defined in either ICD-9-CM or CPT-4.[5] Rehabilitation patient descriptors, such as health status or when and if the patient was discharged from a hospital for the condition under outpatient treatment, also may be important predictors of resource consumption. As a consequence, it is important to consider the use of additional patient level variables that might characterize patient conditions better than is possible using the existing ICD-9-CM or CPT-4 codes. In turn, this may have the effect of improving the APG classification system because APGs are dependent on these two coding systems.

Additional data also might be useful in distinguishing between visits to the emergency room and visits to the outpatient department. The latter are classified into a medical APG. For emergency room visits, certain patient variables, such as the patient's temperature and the patient's living situation, may be important predictors of resources consumed during the visit. This information is not currently collected in either ICD-9-CM or CPT-4.

The research discussed in this chapter had the following objectives:

- To identify a discrete set of clinical signs, symptoms, or findings not currently collected on the UB-92 claim form, or used in ICD-9-CM or CPT-4, that could improve the ability of specific APGs to predict resource consumption.
- To collect a sample of outpatient data with the additional data elements and test the extent to which the additional data improves the ability of specific APGs to predict resource consumption.

STUDY DESIGN

This study involved the collection of information not included on the standard claim form from a variety of clinical settings over a 6-month period. The additional information consists of patient characteristics thought to be useful in improving the ability of APGs to predict resource consumption.

This study is non-random and non-representative and, as such, is not meant to be definitive. It is a starting point for further research. The testing of the proposed diagnosis code modifications was performed in many sites in New York State in conjunction with the New York Department of Health (NYDOH). New York was chosen because much work has been done by NYDOH to better understand outpatient services.

The specific hypothesis tested in this portion of the study was as follows: patient characteristics, such as functional health status, predict resource consumption of outpatient rehabilitation health services over a 1-month period.

Site Selection and Data Collection Process

Appropriate sites were identified by NYDOH personnel and were varied in terms of ownership and types of patient served. For example, in the area of mental health, both private and public, managed care and nonmanaged care sites were sought. NYDOH representatives contacted the institutions to determine their level of interest.

If a site expressed an interest in the project, representatives from NYDOH and 3M Health Information Systems presented to both the site's clinical and administrative staff the purpose and the mechanics of the data collection process. If the staff continued to express interest in participating in the project, they were trained in the objectives and content of the study. NYDOH staff assisted in all the data collection and processing issues. Additionally, in an effort to maintain a high level of interest in the project, site personnel were provided interim- and post-project presentations of their data.

The following sites participated:

- Private, not-for-profit institutions:
  Rusk Rehabilitation Institute
  State University of New York Upstate Medical Center
  Strong Memorial Hospital
  Lutheran Medical Center
- Publicly funded, state-administered sites:
  Helen Hayes Rehabilitation Institute

Definition and resolution of all issues pertaining to data collection and processing constituted a key administrative project objective. Both claims data and clinic-based data had to be collected and merged. There were challenges associated with each data source. Most sites submitted data that could be analyzed.

Two general data processing issues were applicable to all sites:

- Working with clinical settings and information services at participating sites to determine the formats in which data collected on site would be sent to the NYDOH.
- Working with information services at participating sites to assure that claims data extracts were sent by the institution to the NYDOH in a timely and accurate manner.

Once the data processing issues were resolved, on-site training and data collection began. On-site training used a detailed training manual developed to assist individual sites in collecting the data. The manual includes chapters on project background, H-Codes, examples of how to code data elements, the most frequently asked questions pertaining to the research project, and background scientific articles providing further details.

A newsletter was sent to every participating site bimonthly to encourage commitment to the project. After 4–6 weeks of data collection, initial data were processed and a health professional from NYDOH, 3M/HIS, or both visited each site to provide feedback to clinical and administrative professionals. This was done in an effort to maintain interest in the project and to ensure the highest possible accuracy and completeness in the data items collected. Once the project was completed, 3M/HIS personnel offered to return to sites to provide a summary of data results.

When data collection was completed, claims and clinical data were sent to the NYDOH. Clinical data were transferred, if necessary, from paper to electronic format. The two data streams were then merged and dummy record numbers assigned to replace the patient record numbers. A data tape containing both claims and clinical data was then sent to 3M/HIS.

Development of H-Codes

Each of the variables described below was included in the H-Code chapter for several reasons. Each variable was (1) thought to have a high probability of representing an indication of severity, thus making the reason for visit more difficult to treat and requiring more resources; (2) based on information either routinely collected by health care professionals or familiar to them; and (3) derived, whenever possible, from standardized items already tested in the literature.

Independent and dependent variables considered useful in refining rehabilitation and mental illness APGs were not collected for every visit. This was due to the difficulty of collecting additional information on every visit together with a move toward managed care, which reimburses for services provided over time. While the type of visit (family vs. individual therapy) could be identified on a visit basis, additional patient information was collected monthly. A month was adopted as a "bridge" between an individual visit in traditional fee-for-service and a 1-year period summarized under capitation.

Version 2.0 of the medical APGs uses ICD-9-CM diagnosis and CPT procedure codes. Due to frequent provider change from one visit to the next in the ambulatory medical setting, improvement in the medical APGs was sought at the individual visit level. Because data would have needed to be collected for every visit, a short additional data set for potential refinement of the medical APGs was developed. Similarly, refinements in the medical APGs with specific attention to the emergency room also needed to be performed at the individual visit level. Another short additional data set was developed.

The additional information in the H-Codes completely, yet briefly, describes health services in the areas tested in the project.

Two types of H-Codes were collected: independent and dependent variables. Each category of codes is described with a rationale of why the information was collected.

An important means of establishing the validity of the H-Codes will be to evaluate the internal consistency of the functional status levels across items. Measurement error decreases and reliability increases proportionately with the number of internally consistent distinctions made in the assignment of functional status levels.

Independent Variables

Functional health status and time of discharge from a hospitalization (if any) were chosen as variables.

Functional Health Status. Determination of which domains of functional health status to monitor was challenging. Two measures were studied for possible use: The Patient Evaluation and Conference System (PECS) and the Functional Independence Measure (FIM). A significant amount of research has been performed on both measures.[3,4] The PECS was chosen because it was intended to cover both inpatient and outpatient settings, whereas the FIM covers inpatient settings only. Many different domains were considered for possible use as independent variables.

There are two reasons for including a large number of domains in the final data set. First, no literature was available on which domains were likely to be most useful in predicting resource consumption. Second, the experts consulted for this phase of the project felt that a large number of variables were necessary to be certain that all the appropriate domains were chosen.

Time of Discharge from a Hospital. An example of the relevance of this variable is an individual recently discharged from the hospital for a stroke; the patient may consume more resources than a stroke patient at the same functional status level discharged more than a year ago.

Dependent Variables

The dependent variables included provider cost and equipment cost.

Provider Cost. Provider cost was based on time/patient/month spent by each of the treating therapies (physical, occupational, and speech therapy). Time spent with the patient was converted to dollars based on salaries of therapists in the New York City area. Salary structure was obtained from two of the participating sites—both in the New York City area.

Equipment Cost. Equipment cost was based on equipment used by or given to the patient. Equipment was identified on a monthly basis on the supplemental form by the treating therapist.

DATA ANALYSIS

In the data editing process and analysis framework, data from supplemental encounter forms were merged with data from patient claims. The merge algorithm for rehabilitation services is as follows:

- Dummy record numbers replaced patient record numbers to preserve patient confidentiality.
- A month of patient data was allowed only if a supplemental form was completed during the month. This was done to eliminate any instances in which the supplemental form was misplaced or not completed.
- Patient months without any visits were discarded. This was done to eliminate any instances in which the patient visits were misplaced or not completed.
- The supplemental form completion date and dummy record number were used as the keys to join the patient visit(s) that occurred during the month. This was done to ensure patient services were assigned in a consistent manner to the appropriate supplemental form.
- Patient months with no diagnoses coded were discarded because they could not be used in any analysis.
- Patients for whom disequilibrium or mental illness diagnostic categories were identified as the reason for visit were discarded. This was done for two reasons: disequilibrium was treated at only one institution, and mental illness treatment in a rehabilitation setting was not considered to be part of the rehabilitation portion of this study.

The merge algorithm resulted in patients records being eliminated as described in Table 1. Once the data were edited to be certain that valid data were analyzed, the data were formatted into a variety of reports. Table 2 provides a sample report with actual data.

Table 3 provides final statistical results for the groups that were created after detailed examination of the data in conjunction with clinical input. In Table 4, coefficients of variation, standard deviation, and means are provided for each of the groups that were created after data analysis and clinical input. Figure 1 depicts the relationship between the groups.

Classification Tree

Here, we describe the classification of rehabilitation services and the explanatory power of this classification.

The final model has an r^2 of 0.133 for total visits during one month and an r^2 of 0.195 for total cost during one month. A tree for this model is provided in Figure 1.

TABLE 1. Rehabilitation Edits Count and Logic

Step	Description	Patient Months of Rehabilitation Services	%
1	Identify patients with supplemental form(s) for 1 month.	2365	100.00
2	Eliminate patient months without any visit.	1991	84.19
3	Eliminate patient months during which no rehabilitation diagnostic category was defined.	1946	82.28
4	Eliminate patient months for whom disequilibrium or mental illness diagnostic categories were identified as the reason for visit.	1872	79.15

TABLE 2. Aggregate Report Across Months for Acceptance/Understanding of Disability

		Average Visit Count per Patient per Month				Average Equipment Count per Patient per Month					Cost per Patient per Month			
H-Code	Patient Count	PT	OT	SP	Total Average	PT	OT	SP	Total Average	Per Visit	Staff	Equipment	Total	Group Description
H56-	0	0.00	0.00	0.00	0.00	0.00	0.00	0.00	0.00	0.00	0.00	0.00	0.00	No code
H561	6	5.50	0.00	6.00	5.67	0.25	0.00	0.00	0.17	0.03	170.10	0.00	170.10	Extremely poor
H562	20	6.00	0.00	6.88	6.70	1.50	0.00	0.62	0.80	0.12	201.00	12.65	213.65	Moderately to mildly satisfactory
H563	65	5.43	0.00	6.41	6.31	0.14	0.00	0.55	0.51	0.08	189.30	8.00	197.30	Mostly satisfactory
H564	31	3.83	0.00	5.80	5.42	0.00	0.00	0.96	0.77	0.14	162.60	3.19	165.79	Good

H-Code: The H-Code specified in the supplementary code. H56- refers to the supplementary forms for which no code in this domain was checked off.
Patient Count: The number of months of patient visits for which a supplmentary form was coded. This is derived from the claims form.
Average Visit Count Per Patient Per Month: The average number of visits per patient for a month of services for physical therapy (PT), occupational therapy (OT) or speech therapy (SP). This is derived from the claims form.
Total Average: The averages for each treating therapy are averaged to arrive at a total average. This is derived from the claim form.
Average Equipment Count Per Patient Per Month: The number of pieces of equipment used during a month of services for either PT, OT, or SP services. The specific items were checked off by treating therapists at the time of completion of the supplementary form.
Total Average Equipment Per Patient Per Month: The average equipment count per month used in all three therapies.
Per Visit: The average equipment count used in a patient visit.
Cost Per Patient Per Month: Divided into Staff, Equipment, and Total.
Group Descriptions: The level of functional status for that particular domain (acceptance/understanding of disability). The level ranges from extremely poor to good.

TABLE 3. Rehabilitation Statistics for Grouping Structure

		Average Visit Count per Patient per Month				Average Equipment Count per Patient per Month					Cost per Patient per Month			
Group	Patient Count	PT	OT	SP	Total Average	PT	OT	SP	Total Average	Per Visit	Staff	Equipment	Total	Group Description
1	74	5.56	7.80	7.11	6.45	6.00	8.40	3.54	5.39	0.84	193.50	99.84	293.34	Quadriplegia and with feeding problems
2	188	4.97	5.25	6.13	5.66	2.45	1.25	0.60	1.31	0.23	169.80	24.74	194.54	Quadriplegia and without feeding problems
3	198	3.51	4.72	4.34	4.03	1.76	2.44	0.48	1.19	0.29	120.90	13.34	134.24	Hemiplegia, above-knee amputation, complicated fracture with acceptance of disability
4	211	4.01	5.10	5.35	4.89	2.00	1.20	0.88	1.27	0.26	146.70	17.90	164.60	Hemiplegia, above-knee amputation, complicated fracture and without acceptance of disability
5	158	3.82	5.69	5.33	4.78	2.03	4.85	1.01	1.72	0.36	143.40	27.10	170.50	Hemiplegia, above-knee amputation, complicated fracture and with ability to prepare light meal and recent hospital discharge
6	64	6.00	9.33	8.42	8.22	3.73	3.73	5.37	4.70	0.57	246.60	95.44	342.04	Hemiplegia, above-knee amputation, complicated fracture and without recent hospital discharge and with ability to prepare light meal
7	514	2.58	2.15	3.40	2.67	1.98	2.14	0.85	1.71	0.64	80.10	20.51	100.61	Paraplegia, burns, pain, simple fracture and with acceptance
8	305	2.97	3.42	3.91	3.25	2.85	3.36	0.97	2.43	0.75	97.50	40.40	138.00	Paraplegia, burns, pain, simple fracture and without acceptance
9	98	2.76	1.86	4.66	3.32	1.53	1.71	0.78	1.30	0.39	99.60	21.07	120.67	Paraplegia, burns, pain, simple fracture with recent hospital discharge with ability to prepare light meal
10	62	4.47	6.73	8.89	5.66	5.11	2.00	6.22	4.52	0.80	169.80	92.73	262.53	Paraplegia, burns, pain, simple fracture and with recent hospital discharge and and without ability to prepare light meal

(group 10). Similar patients who could prepare a light meal consumed \$120 per month (group 9). Patients who did not have recent hospitalization but did have an acceptance or understanding of the disability consumed \$138 per month of rehabilitative services (group 8), while the patients who did not have an acceptance or understanding of the disability consumed \$100 of rehabilitative services per month (group 7).

The coefficients of variation for the different rehabilitation groups are provided in Table 4. The relatively low CVs (ranging from 0.53–0.96) emanate from the relatively tight (0.65–1.31) distribution of staff costs. The group (group 10) with relatively high CV (1.31) had only 62 patients. There is considerable variation in equipment costs (with CVs from 0.8–2.5) with several categories having patient months with minimal to no equipment costs. The question of reliable coding of equipment use arises in categories having patient months with no equipment costs.

Rasch analyses of data from different functional assessment instruments and different samples of patients, recorded at different facilities by different therapists and by the patients themselves, reveals the extent to which these instruments measure the same thing.[1] Research aimed at taking advantage of these common structures formally equates the instruments in order to deploy a universal, scale-free metric unit of measurement for each variable.[2]

Although formal study of the H-Code data has yet to be completed, initial Rasch analysis results indicate general agreement with the results of prior studies of similar instruments, such as the PECS and the FIM. H-Code domains are the most similar to the PECS Motor Skills and Community Reintegration scales.[6] The 16 domains in the D-Code version of the Community Reintegration scale have a measurement reliability of 0.84. Both scales have satisfactory statistical consistency in the order of the items over the persons measured and vice versa.

Further research will determine the extent to which the H-Code scales can be equated with other scales ostensibly measuring the same variables. Should it then be possible to satisfactorily predict health service resource consumption using these and other measures, the H-Codes could be generated automatically from reference tables or by computer, averting unnecessary duplication of functional health status data. Further work will show how the scale-free metrics could be integrated into the APG framework.

DISCUSSION

This study attempted to identify a discrete set of variables that might improve the ability of several types of APGs to predict resource consumption for rehabilitation services.

In particular, this study examined the hypothesis that selected patient characteristics, such as diagnosis and aspects of functional status, correlate with resource consumption of rehabilitation health services over a 1-month period. Resource consumption was defined here as a combination of rehabilitation treatment therapies and equipment cost.

Diagnosis alone, a patient characteristic already collected on the claim form, has an r^2 of 0.092. This is not surprising because many diagnoses, such as quadriplegia, include aspects of functional status within the diagnosis itself. However, the inclusion of additional elements, such as time since hospital discharge, if any, and aspects of functional status, improve the r^2 to 0.14 for total visits and 0.195 for total cost for 1 month. At the same time, functional health status measurement is familiar to most providers of rehabilitation services. Many institutions already collect this type of information regularly. Further research on larger groups of patients is necessary to evaluate the impact of specific aspects of functional status that could not be assessed for lack of a large enough data set.

CONCLUSION

This prospective study represents the first time selected patient characteristics were used to predict resource consumption for rehabilitation health services over a short time. This work is particularly important at a time of significantly increased interest in managed care. This study also represents the first effort to quantify the relationship between selected patient characteristics and case management time.

Results of this study heighten the importance of a better understanding of the relationship between patient characteristics and resource consumption of health services. The current push to managed care mandates more research to increase our understanding of the determinants of resource consumption in health services. This study begins the process of understanding the relationship between resource consumption and patient characteristics for patients whose consumption of resources has been historically difficult to understand using data available from a claim form.

RECOMMENDATIONS

On the basis of work summarized in this report several recommendations could be considered:

- For certain services, such as rehabilitation, the Health Care Financing Administration could consider a demonstration project that would evaluate payment for outpatient mental health services or rehabilitation services using a quasicapitated methodology based on the variables collected in this study. The research summarized in this chapter could provide a methodologic approach and represent a bridge between fee-for-service and managed care. There are carve-outs for managed care of rehabilitation services, and thus a similar project would have relevance to today's health care market.
- An important follow-up research project could examine the patient characteristics that would predict resource consumption of inpatient and outpatient rehabilitation or mental health services. This project would complete the bridge between fee-for-service and managed care. Such a research project would examine the costs of services for stroke patients in the outpatient, inpatient, and nursing home setting.
- Application of scale-free measurement models to functional health status data stands to improve the quality of these data and to make them easier to use. Because of the high stakes involved in applications of functional assessment (data systems, quality of care comparisons, accreditation, research), extra effort should be made to take advantage of scale-free measurement's routine evaluations of data quality, transformation of ordinal ratings into interval measures, and equating of different brands of instruments shown to measure the same thing.

REFERENCES

1. Fisher WP Jr, Harvey RF, Kilgore KM: New developments in functional assessment: Probabilistic models for gold standards. Neurorehabilitation 5:3–25, 1995.
2. Fisher WP Jr, Harvey RF, Taylor P, et al: Rehabits: A common language of functional assessment. Arch Phys Med Rehabil 76:113–122, 1995.
3. Hamilton BB, Granger CV, Sherwin FS, et al: A uniform national data system for medical rehabilitation. In Fuhrer MJ (ed): Rehabilitation Outcomes Analysis and Measurement. Baltimore, Brookes, 1987.

4. Harvey RF, Jellinek HM: Functional performance assessment: A program approach. Arch Phys Med Rehabil 62:456–461, 1981.
5. Jencks SF, Hogan C, Goldman HH, Taube CA: Bringing excluded psychiatric facilities under the Medicare prospective payment system. A review of research evidence and policy options. Med Care 25, 1987.
6. Kilgore KM, Fisher WP Jr, Silverstein B, et al: Application of Rasch analysis to the patient evaluation and conference system. Phys Med Rehabil Clin North Am 4:493–515, 1993.

WILLIAM P. FISHER, JR, PHD

WHAT SCALE-FREE MEASUREMENT MEANS TO OUTCOMES RESEARCH

From the Department of Public Health and Preventive Medicine
Louisiana State University School of Medicine
Louisiana State University Medical Center
New Orleans, Louisiana

Reprint requests to:
William P. Fisher, Jr, PhD
Louisiana State University Medical Center
School of Medicine in New Orleans
1600 Canal Street–Room 809
New Orleans, LA 70112

"There is nothing more difficult to plan, more doubtful of success, nor more dangerous to manage than the creation of a new system. For the initiator has the enmity of all who would profit by the preservation of the old institutions, and merely lukewarm defenders in those who should gain by the new ones."

—Machiavelli

"A new scientific truth does not triumph by convincing its opponents and making them see the light but rather because its opponents eventually die, and a new generation grows up that is familiar with it."

—Max Planck

"There are three stages to the life of revolutionary scientific ideas. They are initially rejected as outrageous heresies, then they are recognized as brilliant discoveries, and finally they are assumed to be the way things have always been."

—William James (paraphrased)

The history of measurement is tightly intertwined with the history of economics. The history of British weights and measures, for instance, shows that metrological systems proliferate during periods of economic depression dominated by local trade, whereas widely accepted metrological standards emerge in periods of economic expansion characterized by regional and international trade.[40]

The economic transformation of health care taking place today thus has many historical precedents. We are moving from local economies of disease-crisis management to a global economy of preventive health management. As the effort to shift the focus of health care from disease management to health management gets underway, the need to compare health status (physical and psychosocial functioning, quality of life and life satisfaction, risk behaviors, and satisfaction with services) across groups, regionally, nationally, and internationally, increases.

The problem is that the transformation of the system cannot take place as long as health status is measured in scale-dependent units that vary in their size and meaning by instrument brand, provider, plan, and patient, and in the presence of missing data. The most commonly proffered solution to this problem is to have all users employ the same scale and always supply complete data, which at least offers the appearance that the same thing is measured. A number of data-sharing schemes based on common scale use have emerged (HEDIS, FOTO, CROA, Medirisk, UDS), but these are flawed in a number of ways, including their need for complete data, their incapacity to adapt to the needs of individuals, their lack of data quality control, their treatment of ordinal data as interval, their lack of individual error estimates for each measure, and their mutual incommensurability.

Scale-free measurement models[2–4,22–24,28,29,35–37,39] overcome all of these problems. As it becomes increasingly clear that the accountability of educators, psychologists, health care providers, and other professionals cannot remain tied to local indicators incapable of supporting evidence-based decision-making and evaluation, the practicality, scientific rigor, and mathematical beauty of scale-free measurement will become more widely appreciated. Furthermore, as the computational capacity to implement accountability measures, and the telecommunications capacity to implement wide-scale comparisons mount hand-in-hand, the intellectual and methodologic skills required to use scale-free measurement techniques will become automated. Taken together with the economic demand for accountability and comparisons, these factors will eventually make scale-free measurement commonplace.

CREATION AND IMPLEMENTATION OF SCALE-FREE OUTCOME MEASURES

Recent social studies of laboratory science have led some to the opinion that social scientists have ignored or devalued the role of social networks in the creation of scientific objectivity, generality, and laws. For instance, O'Connell says, "The challenge to social scientists is to stop taking the universality of entities like the volt for granted, and to start treating the volt like the *society* which it truly is—a distributed collective connected by continually renewed structured relations of exchange and authority. Scientific entities are not universal until scientists or their technicians take the trouble to make them so."[26] O'Connell seems to be saying that the problem for social scientists is recognizing that physical scientists do not have any special epistemologic advantages that accrue from a supposedly natural objectivity associated with the phenomena studied. The implication is that social scientists do not take the trouble to make the entities they study universal because they have not set up the required social networks.

Similarly, Widmalm says, "Technical reliability depends on the organization of people. Scientific conventions, such as standards, are both agents of unity and products of agreement . . . . The adoption of standards reflects the adoption of laboratory cultures. Precision is the result not only of individual technical prowess, but of networks of scientists who rely on an infrastructure of workshops and bureaucracies."[34] And Schaffer says, "The physical values which the laboratory fixes are sustained by the social values which the laboratory inculcates . . . . In milieux such as those of Victorian Britain the propagation of standards and values was the means through which physicists reckoned they could link their work with technical and economic projects elsewhere in their society. Instrumental ensembles let these workers embody the values which mattered to their culture in their laboratory routines. Intellectualist condescension distracts our attention from these everyday practices, from their technical staff, and from the work which makes results count outside laboratory walls."[30] Even in the field of historical metrology, "weights and measures officials are almost never discussed, and if they are they receive only brief mention as a footnote to a presentation of the units."[40]

But are epistemologic naiveté and intellectualist condescension toward everyday practices and social organization the only reasons why social scientists have not succeeded in establishing the scientific universality of the entities they study? Probably not, as at least some leaders in the social sciences have not succumbed to these failings. There are, for instance, many dozens of professional associations of social scientists. The annual meetings of these groups bring together quoting circles and participants in research traditions who share a great deal in the way of convention and standards.

So what is missing in the everyday practices and social organization of the social sciences, roughly defined as areas of study that employ rating scales or tests as the instruments of measurement? What prevents the social sciences from discovering and inventing mathematical laws of human behavior, attitudes, and knowledge? More specifically, why do the social sciences lack universally accepted metrics for measuring their variables of interest? Various answers to these questions come to mind. First, scale-free measurement research to date has focused mostly on the creation of models, the derivation of efficient estimation algorithms, methods for evaluating model fit, and software development. Second, most applications of this work have taken place within the traditional scale-dependent orientation to data analysis and the interpretation of results, meaning that generalization has typically stopped far short of the kinds of statements that fit to a scale-free model can support. Third, most social scientists are unaware of, or untrained in, the scale-free measurement theories and methods that would make universal units of measurement possible. Finally, users, standards groups, and the general public are unaware of scale-free measurement and its potential for improving communication, efficiency, and effectiveness in education and health care.

Several networks for sharing information on outcomes of care in common formats are emerging, but none has yet taken the step of expressing health status, quality of life, satisfaction with services, or the propensity to risk health in scale-free metrics. It seems that scale-free measurement and the health care outcomes information communities need to join together to form a consensus on the structure and content of these metrics. A suggested course of action has three components: (1) gather and publicize evidence supporting the existence of scale-free measurement structures; (2) involve users in the creation of the networks through which universal metrological standards will be implemented and monitored; and (3) form a new association of professionals who share scale-free measurement values, so that the needed evidence can be assembled and publicized with the credibility such an association can provide. These themes are explored below.

The Need for Evidence

The need for the most basic kinds of education regarding measurement principles is evident in reviewers' comments on and criticisms of grant applications and article submissions. For instance, one reviewer of a Rasch-measurement based health status study proposal comments: "The application asserts that 'in order for a measure of health status to be consistently structured and validly measured, the probable order of the items on the measuring instrument, as determined by the sum of their ratings across respondents, should not vary in a manner that depends on who is measured.' This statement appears to deny the possibility that health status may indeed vary depending on an individual's characteristics. On these grounds, the basic premise of the research is questionable." This reviewer has missed the distinction between denying the possibility of variation in health status item order and exploring the extent to which invariance holds across or within groups. The same reviewer says: "The application does not explain how the hypotheses will be tested. In fact, it is not clear that some are even testable. For example, 'health status can be quantified more rigorously, with a lower error of measurement, higher reliability, and better model fit, than is currently achieved by existing health status instruments.' How can one test whether measure A is better than measure B . . . without having some standard against which to compare both? When both measures rely on the same technique—a questionnaire—both are simply windows on the same unobservable construct." It is evident that the reviewer is not qualified to evaluate the proposal, as she or he has no grasp of fundamental measurement concepts.

Reviewers constantly repeat that Rasch methods require detailed and simple introductions, precluding presentation of detailed or complex analyses, even after 5 or 10 introductory articles have appeared in the journal in question. For instance, even after one physical medicine and rehabilitation journal published at least 10 articles employing Rasch measurement, reviewers still refer to Rasch models as statistical models being fit to data (instead of as measurement models to which data are fit); admit ignorance regarding Rasch-based model fit, reliability indices, and the logic of item anchoring; and then state that "I'm not sure whether the analysis and interpretation was performed by someone who knew what they were doing." When the article was resubmitted with an Acknowledgments section detailing the five different Rasch and other meetings at which the analyses were presented, the editor mailed the original of the reviewer's comments to the author, apparently to clear the editor of any responsibility for the mistakes in the review.

Another reviewer in the same journal states in reference to another submission that "Believability is stretched a bit by the notion that there is an *invariant* order of pain complaint's frequency from one patient to another, . . . [although, apparently,] the author is not at all surprised by this."

These reviewers' comments reveal that there is a need for demonstrations not only of item invariance across patient samples, but of *construct* invariance across instruments intended to measure the same variable, when these are applied to common and different samples. At least two studies document health status variable stability over diagnostic-related groups for single instruments.[15,18] Several studies document health status or quality of life construct invariance across instruments.[8–12] Examination of the results of the application of scale-free measurement models to data from other health status instruments[13,31] suggests that these also address the same construct in the same metric or a linearly transformable version of it. The figures demonstrate the sample-free quality of one instrument's item calibrations.

Sample Evidence: Functional Independence Measure Item Calibrations

Work recently completed at the Louisiana Rehabilitation Institute (LRI) in New Orleans compares the published calibrations for a health status instrument with calibrations estimated from a local sample but not included in the published study.[25,27] Figure 1 shows a plot of admission and discharge Rasch calibrations of all 18 of the

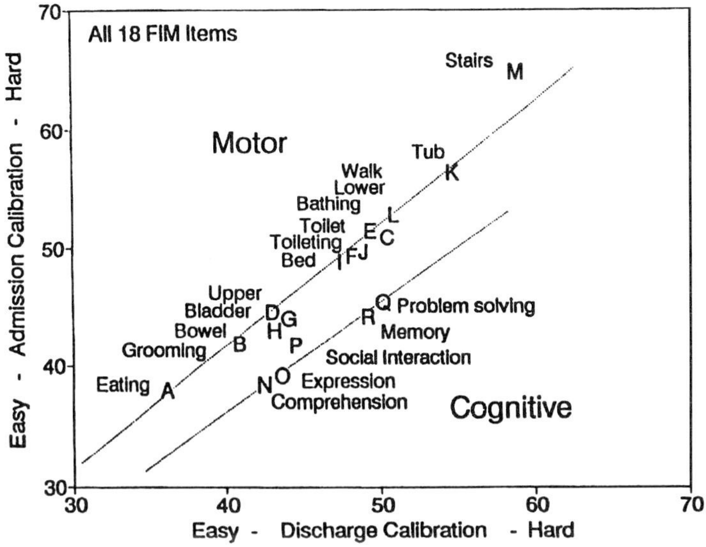

FIGURE 1. Comparison of FIM Admission and Discharge Calibrations. (From Wright BD, Linacre JM, Heinemann AW: Measuring functional status in rehabilitation. Phys Med Rehabil Clin North Am 4:475–491, 1993; with permission.)

Functional Independence Measure (FIM) items.[38] The data were from the Uniform Data System (UDS) and included more than 25,000 patients. Figure 2 shows another plot of admission and discharge Rasch calibrations of all 18 of the FIM items. This time the data are from 72 patients admitted to the LRI in 1994 and 1995. The 72 patients are neither in the UDS database nor included in the analysis of Wright et al.[38] or Linacre et al.[19] However, the motor and cognitive items line up on their different slopes in almost identical patterns.

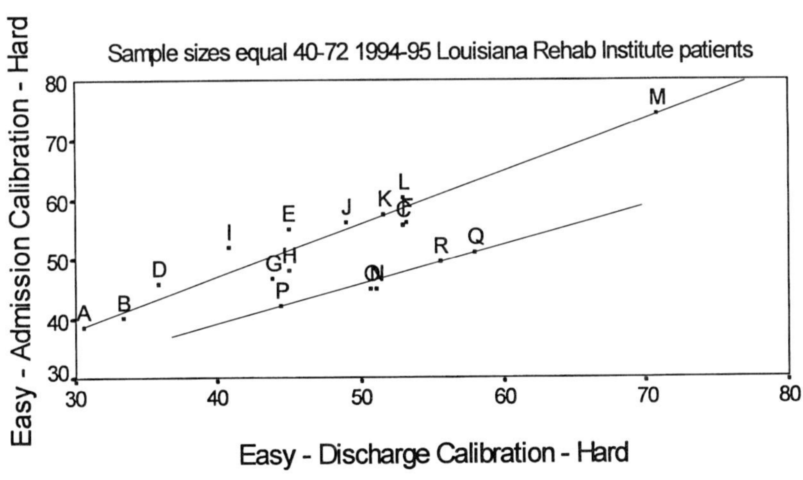

FIGURE 2. Comparison of Louisiana Rehabilitation Institute Functional Independence Measure admit and discharge calibrations (18 items).

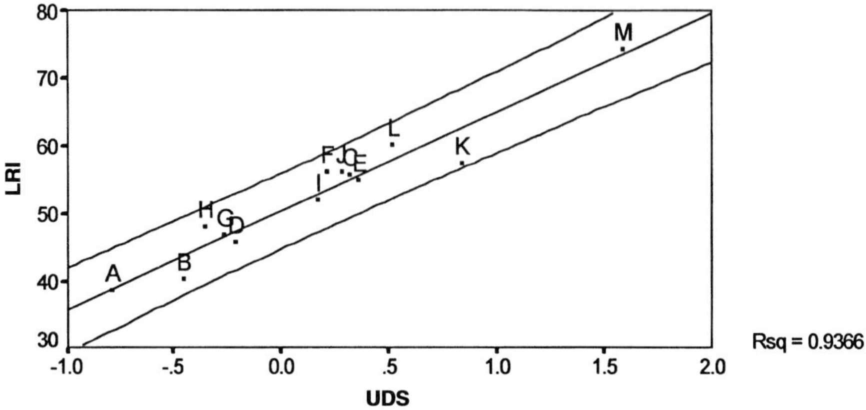

FIGURE 3. Comparison of Louisiana Rehabilitation Institute and UDS Functional Independence Measure motor skills scales. Admission FIM motor skills.

Figures 3–6 plot the LRI and UDS admission and discharge data by scale. The admission motor skills data (Fig. 3) produce an R-square of 0.94, and the discharge motor skills scales (Fig. 4) have an R-square of 0.83; both are high enough to say the variable is stable across the samples.

The two cognitive skills scale plots (Figs. 5 and 6) display an anomaly—one apparent in the LRI combined-scale plot. In contrast with the UDS's cognitive skills scale, the LRI's places item P, social interaction, at the bottom of the measurement continuum, as the easiest item on the scale and the one most likely to provoke high ratings. A possible explanation is revealed by the consideration of the patients' ICD9 diagnostic codes in relation to the documented diagnostic-group variations found in the FIM cognitive skills scale item calibration.[15]

Heinemann shows that, for patients suffering a stroke on the right side of the brain, social interaction rests at the bottom, easy end of the scale with auditory comprehension, verbal expression being almost as difficult as memory for these persons.[15]

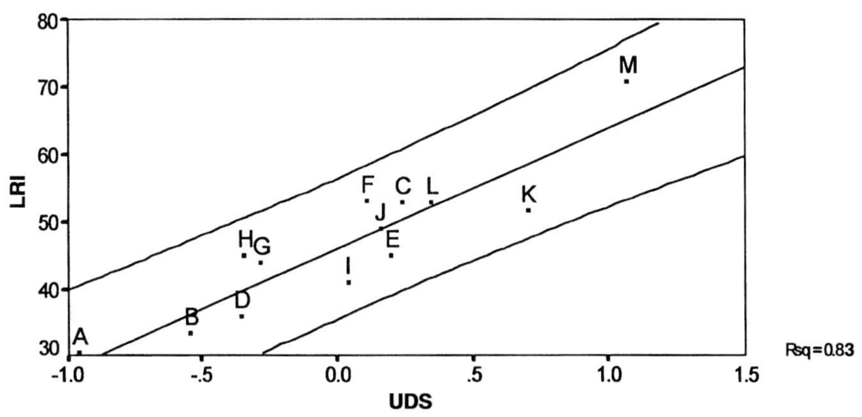

FIGURE 4. Comparison of Louisiana Rehabilitation Institute and UDS motor skills scales. Discharge FIM motor skills. Sample size = 25,000. LRI sample size = 70.

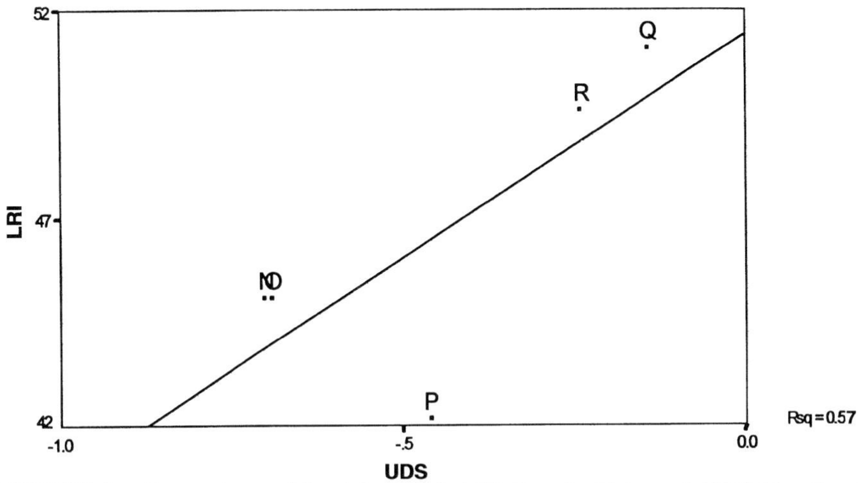

FIGURE 5. Comparison of Louisiana Rehabilitation Institute and UDS Functional Independence Measure cognitive skills scales. Admission FIM cognition scale.

At least 42 of the 70 LRI patients have an ICD9 code in their medical record indicating cerebrovascular accident, but how many of these occurred on the right side of the brain is unclear. If the matter is related to the predominance of stroke victims in the LRI sample, further investigation should also look into why auditory comprehension is as difficult as verbal expression for the LRI patients, and not as easy as social interaction, as it is for the UDS right CVA sample.

When a small proportion of items in a scale change position in a sample-dependent manner, the common metric is not threatened as long as enough items share common scale values to provide a stable structure for equating. The items that vary in difficulty are treated as addressing different aspects of the construct in ways especially

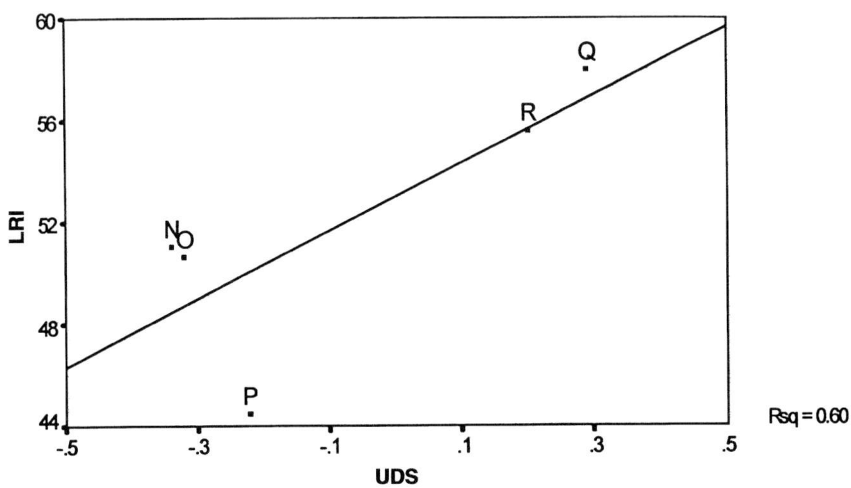

FIGURE 6. Comparison of Louisiana Rehabilitation Institute and UDS Functional Independence Measure cognitive skills scales. Discharge FIM cognition scale.

relevant to the different samples. Should most or all items change their scale values across samples by more than two errors, there is no common construct. This apparently negative result has the positive effect of provoking recognition of differences that might otherwise be glossed over, probably to the detriment of one or both groups.

Implications and Next Steps

The research on the equating of instruments intended to measure physical functioning[9–11,16] and comparisons of independently conducted calibration studies[13,15,18,31] strongly suggests that the construct is stable across a range of instruments, diagnostic groups, health care providers, and geographic regions. Further research will establish the extent to which the physical functioning and other health status, quality of life, risk behavior, and satisfaction with service variables can each be expressed in universal metrics.

Beyond the research, universal implementation of scale-free metrics will require the cooperation and understanding of the many groups that will use them. Implementation also will require mechanisms for monitoring, maintaining, and improving data quality. Many kinds of measurement systems mandated by federal and state regulatory agencies are out of statistical control.[6,17] Even when the quality of a measurement system is monitored, the monitors are sometimes poorly conceived or executed. Poorly designed or controlled measuring systems exist in every field, with huge economic consequences. In the late 1970s it was estimated that physical measurement activities made up 6% of the U.S. gross national product and that the indirect cost of uncontrolled measurement systems must be several times that.[17]

These estimates do not include the plethora of uncontrolled and idiosyncratically instrument- and sample-dependent measures in widespread use in medicine, education, psychology, and the social sciences. Rigorously designed and executed research in these fields has produced results that are not strikingly less consistent than results from the physical sciences,[14] but the quality of measures in general classroom and clinic use is unknown. Supplanting local, incommensurable, and uncontrolled systems with quality assessed and improved scale-free metric systems will take time and effort, with a return on the investment that will go beyond mere dollars to tangible improvements in the quality of life for many.

IMPLEMENTING AND MONITORING UNIVERSAL METRICS

American Society for Testing and Materials

Models of, and a place for, a network of measurement technicians and users interested in implementing and monitoring scale-free measurement standards exist in the American Society for Testing and Materials (ASTM), an organization with a long history of developing and disseminating standards according in interested parties' criteria and input. The ASTM electronic medical record subcommittee, formally known as Subcommittee E31.19 on the Vocabulary for Computer-Based Patient Record Content and Structure, has expressed interest in Rasch's models for scale-free measurement, as these stand to offer unique advantages for rating scale data quality control, quantification, and outcomes comparison. The head of the E31.19 subcommittee has invited all interested parties to contribute their expertise to the development of quality and quantity standards for medical outcomes data. A working group on rating scale measurement standards for the electronic medical record has been established within ASTM committee E31.19.

The ASTM Health Care Informatics Standards Committee E31, of which the E31.19 subcommittee is a part, has released a review of published standards and current projects that the includes the following description of ASTM:

> ASTM was organized in 1898 and has grown into one of the largest voluntary standards development systems in the world. It is a not-for-profit organization that provides a forum for producers, users, ultimate consumers, and those having a general interest to meet on common neutral ground and write standards for materials, products, systems, and services. From the work of 134 standards-writing committees, ASTM publishes more than 8,500 standards in 68 volumes of the Annual Book of ASTM Standards. These standards cover a wide variety of subject areas, and the work is done voluntarily by 33,000 technically qualified ASTM members in over 80 countries around the world.
>
> ASTM provides a number of services to its technical committees:
>
> - It provides a management system, known as a full consensus process, that has been refined and proven to be a reliable way to produce useful acceptable standards. This process involves several levels of balloting, strict mechanisms to ensure all viewpoints are considered, and protection against domination by any single interest group.
> - A staff manager is assigned to work with each committee to provide a central point of contact for the public, handle most of the administrative details, and provide guidance on ASTM procedures and policy.
> - ASTM publishes the standards, handles the publicity about them, and provides a point of sale for people who need them.
> - ASTM provides its members protection from liability.
>
> About 85% of ASTM's income is from the sale of publications. This includes the standards, five journals, and numerous peer-reviewed special technical publications. Besides writing and publishing standards, ASTM sponsors symposia, technical and professional training sessions, and other educational activities.
>
> ASTM has been active in medical computing because professionals and others working in this area have found it to be a suitable home in which to develop standards. The typical participants are experts with an appreciation of how things might be better in their particular disciplines if standards could be agreed upon. Often ASTM works in concert with relevant professional societies and other related organizations. This helps ensure the standards are responsive to the needs of the whole industry and are not duplicative of another group's work. In the area of health care informatics, ASTM was a founding member of the Health Care Informatics Standards Planning Panel within the American National Standards Institute (ANSI). ASTM Committee 31 is committed to cooperation with other standards writing bodies so that the various standards will converge to a useful result rather than diverge into various incompatible protocols.

This statement suggests that the ASTM is a place in which the viability of Rasch's models for measurement as means for creating and maintaining scale-free standards can be publicly tested, evaluated, and established in a fair and open forum. It also seems that the values of the ASTM standards committees' members and Rasch measurement practitioners regarding measurement quality and the need for universally available and understood quantities are quite alike.

In a paper entitled "Evolving with Technology: Information Systems, Standards, and Public Health," the Joint Council of Governmental Public Health Agencies (JCGPHA) reviews current health-related standards development activities. In response to the question, "What is a standard?", this paper states:

> Standardization refers to the general acceptance of concepts, quantities, terms, rules, and definitions that serve as reference points for professionals in a given field.

> Standards provide criteria for a common language, ensuring reliable communication between all parties in the conduct of business. For example, U.S. electrical current standards, which cover voltage, amperage, outlets, and plugs, are so widely accepted that manufacturers automatically incorporate them into their designs. These standards streamline product development for manufacturers and ensure consumers hassle-free usage regardless of where they live in the U.S. or what type of appliance they purchase. Standardization also permits government regulatory agencies to ensure product safety.
>
> In the context of health-related data and information systems, necessary standards include, among others: standardized definitions; standards for the context of data sets; standards for electronic transmission of data; standards for aggregation; and uniform patient, provider, and payer identifiers. General acceptance of these standards will ensure the comparability of data, allowing information to be aggregated and analyzed for performance assessment and epidemiological studies. Standards also allow data to be shared across the multitude of public health providers and managed care systems, which help to ensure continuity in patient care management and reduction in duplicative services. Used smartly, data standards will go a long way toward decreasing costs and confusion in the health system.

Electrical current standards make the use of electrical appliances "hassle-free" in that consumers are liberated from concerns regarding the physical and mechanical configurations of the machines. Any machine will operate reliably no matter which outlet it is plugged into across a wide geographic range. Conversely, any outlet will provide the correct receptacle and amount of current for any relevant machine. This kind of "machine-free" outlet voltage provision and "outlet-free" machine voltage consumption corresponds with the Rasch measurement sense of "sample-free" instrument calibration and "scale-free" person measurement.[36] The economic effects of scale-free measurement will surely be on a scale equaling or exceeding the effects of standards in the materials sciences.

Conducting Equating Studies

The JCGPHA paper points out that work done by ASTM and other groups has not made public health's information needs a priority, and so nothing on health status, preventive services, or health outcomes has been included in the standards documents. However, the July 1995 revision of the ASTM E31.19 subcommittee report E1384-91, "A Standard Guide for Content and Structure of the Computer Based Patient Report," includes database fields for admission and discharge 18-item FIM scores, for Rancho cognitive level scores, and for a patient-generated functional health status score.

The only alternatives to scale-dependent ordinal scores mentioned by the JCGPHA paper are uniform data sets in which each data element is a nominal category, and no effort at aggregation, scoring, or measurement is made. Similarly, the ASTM expectation has been that there would be no alternative but to accept particular scales' ordinal metrics as standard content in the computerized medical record. But both the ordinal and the nominal data systems omit crucial data quality checks; have rigid, stifling data completeness requirements; achieve only the appearance of information standardization; and offer no framework informed by construct studies, additive measures, error estimates, or fit analysis in which to interpret the meaning of the data available. All of these problems could be overcome with scale-free measurement techniques, which share much in common with standard ASTM statistical methods for determining measurement precision and consistency.

Although concerned primarily with physical measurements, ASTM publications on the within-laboratory repeatability and between-laboratory reproducibility of measurement methods are analogous to Rasch measurement practitioners' concerns with data consistency, model fit, the variation/error or signal/noise reliability ratio (separation), and multifaceted designs.[20,21,32,33] Rasch-calibrated variable stability is evaluated by comparing item calibrations from different samples of respondents and by comparing person measures from different item samples. Similarly, the ASTM standard practice for conducting an interlaboratory study to determine the precision of a test method is intended to establish that instruments intended to measure the same thing actually do[5] and that they do so to comparable degrees of precision.

In ASTM parlance, repeatability and reproducibility measures capture the opposite extremes of precision. Repeatability studies exclude from consideration local factors that can influence measurement precision, such as the person operating the equipment, the particular equipment used, the equipment's calibration, and environmental conditions such as temperature, humidity, and air quality. Reproducibility studies include these factors and evaluate their influence on variable stability. Typical results show that precision varies more across operators or across equipment than within the measures produced by a single operator on a single machine.

ASTM standard practice focuses on two statistics in particular: h, the between-laboratory consistency statistic, and k, the within-laboratory consistency statistic. The h statistic is calculated as

$$h = d/s_{\bar{x}} \quad (1)$$

where:

h	=	the between-laboratory consistency statistic,
d	=	the cell deviation (i.e., the deviation of the cell average from the average of the cell averages), and
$s_{\bar{x}}$	=	the standard deviation of the cell averages.

The k statistic is calculated as

$$k = s/s_r \quad (2)$$

where:

k	=	the within-laboratory consistency statistic,
s	=	the cell standard deviation for one laboratory, and
s_r	=	the repeatability standard deviation of the material.

ASTM standard practice employs these statistics in graphs to study measures across and within laboratories[5] to evaluate measurement precision and to determine whether the system is under statistical control. In the clinician-awarded rating scale measurement context, the h and k statistics could be calculated on measures made on common samples circulated among facilities participating in the common metric; these samples would be text, video, or multimedia presentations of persons with commonly found impairments and disabilities. In the contexts of both clinician-awarded ratings and self-reported ratings, the h and k statistics and graphs would also be used to understand the consistency of the calibrations obtained from commonly employed items on independent samples. Scale values for all sample individuals with multiple measures, and for all items with multiple calibrations, from different facilities, would also be studied by plotting differences between pairs of scale values against their means,[1,7] as has been done by Cella, Fisher, and their colleagues.[10,12] The usual Rasch approach to variable stability analysis, plotting pairs of scale values together,[23,39] should also be employed for visual confirmation of their relationship.

The advantage of the h and k statistics is that interpretation of interlaboratory measurement precision consistency is aided by the availability of critical values for each at the the 0.50% significance level, for data from 3–30 laboratories.[5] Three significance levels have been evaluated by ASTM. The 0.50% level was chosen because 1.00% was too sensitive, flagging too many cells as inconsistent, and because 0.10% was too insensitive, flagging too few cells for examination. Data from at least six laboratories are recommended for sufficient power.

Having begun with the plotted scale values in the above examples using the FIM values shown in Table 1, we can continue by calculating the h consistency statistics for the different calibrations. Treating the items as "materials" and the distinct calibrations as "laboratories," each item's calibration estimate, being the average calibration across the steps between adjacent rating categories, substitutes for the cell average used in calculating d in equation (1). Because rating scale models, and not partial credit models, were employed in all four of these calibrations, the standard deviations of the within-laboratory item calibrations are identical, causing the k statistic to be the same with each repetition. For this reason, the k statistic is omitted from the following example.

Figures 7 and 8 show the h statistics for the LRI and UDS admission and discharge FIM calibrations. Figure 7 groups the calibrations ("laboratories") by item,

TABLE 1. Calibration Estimates Used in Figures 2–8

Item Number	Item Name	LINADMC	LINDISC	LRIADMC	LRIDISC	LINADMC2	LINDISC2
1	A. Eating	–0.79	–0.96	38.60	30.60	42.10	40.40
2	B. Grooming	–0.45	–0.54	40.30	33.40	45.50	44.60
3	C. Bathing	0.32	0.24	55.80	53.00	53.20	52.40
4	D. Dressing UE	–0.21	–0.35	45.80	35.90	47.90	46.50
5	E. Dressing LE	0.36	0.20	55.00	45.00	53.60	52.00
6	F. Toileting	0.21	0.11	56.20	53.20	52.10	51.10
7	G. Bladder	–0.26	–0.28	46.80	43.90	47.40	47.20
8	H. Bowel	–0.35	–0.34	48.10	45.00	46.50	46.60
9	I. Bed/Ch/Whchr	0.17	0.04	52.00	40.90	51.70	50.40
10	J. Toilet	0.28	0.16	56.20	49.00	52.80	51.60
11	K. Tub/shower	0.84	0.70	57.60	51.60	58.40	57.00
12	L. Walk	0.52	0.35	60.30	53.00	55.20	53.50
13	M. Stairs	1.59	1.07	74.40	70.80	65.90	60.70
14	N. Compreh	–0.70	–0.34	45.10	51.10	43.00	46.60
15	O. Express	–0.69	–0.32	45.10	50.70	43.10	46.80
16	P. Social inter	–0.46	–0.22	42.20	44.50	45.40	47.80
17	Q. Prob solv	–0.14	0.29	51.10	58.00	48.60	52.90
18	R. Memory	–0.24	0.20	49.60	55.60	47.60	52.00

LINADMC: Admission Calibration. *From Linacre[19]
LINDISC: Discharge Calibration. *From Linacre[19]
LRIADMC: Admission Calibration.
LRIDISC: Discharge Calibration.
LINADMC2: Admission Calibration times 10, and plus 50, for conversion to LRI 0–100 metric. *From Linacre[19]
LINDISC: Discharge Calibration times 10, and plus 50, for conversion to LRI 0–100 metric. *From Linacre[19]

and Figure 8 groups the items by calibration. None of the values indicate statistically significant inconsistency, although many of the LRI values approach the critical values of –1.49 and 1.49. The graphs show that the LRI item calibrations are typically more different from the overall by-item means than the UDS calibrations. Three groups of LRI calibrations can be identified as potentially problematic: the admission and discharge motor skills items (items A–M) and the discharge cognitive skills items (items N–R).

Six of the LRI motor skill and four of the cognitive skill admission calibration items have *h* statistics less than –1.0, indicating that the item calibration was at least one standard deviation greater than the average calibration for that item across laboratories (subtracting each cell average/item calibration from the mean leaves a negative residual for calibrations greater than the mean). Eight of the LRI motor skills discharge calibration items have *h* statistics over 1.0, indicating that the item calibration was at least one standard deviation less than the average calibration for that item across laboratories.

An *h* statistic greater than 1.0 or less than –1.0 is a relatively large difference compared to the differences of the other calibrations from their overall mean, this being established by dividing each cell deviation from their by-item means by the standard deviation of the cell averages. When the standardized differences from the mean (the *h* statistic) is evaluated in terms of the power of the experimental design using Student's *t* and the *F*-ratio, the amount of tolerable deviation increases as the number of laboratories involved increases. Critical values for *h* range from 1.15 with three laboratories to 2.64 with 30.[5] There are larger differences among the critical values for the low-powered designs (those with fewer laboratories) than for the high-powered designs, with the differences being about 0.01 for 18 or more laboratories.

Interestingly, and probably not coincidentally, the larger *h*-values for the LRI FIM item calibrations are associated with these calibrations' lower sample sizes and higher errors. The lack of *h*-values exceeding the critical cutoffs confirms the significance of the correlations among the calibrations. Further experience will enable evaluation of the associations among these design elements and will indicate how they can be used to assess and improve measurement quality.

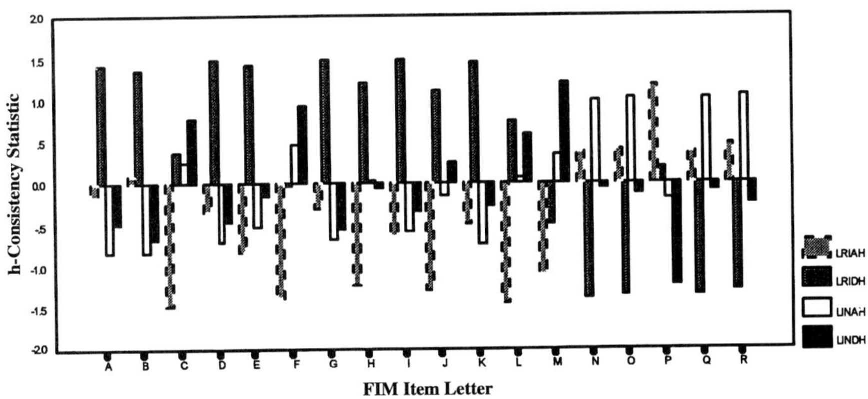

Critical value of h for n of 4 labs at 0.50% significance level = 1.49.
No values are greater than |1.49|.

FIGURE 7. FIM calibrations: Laboratories within items.

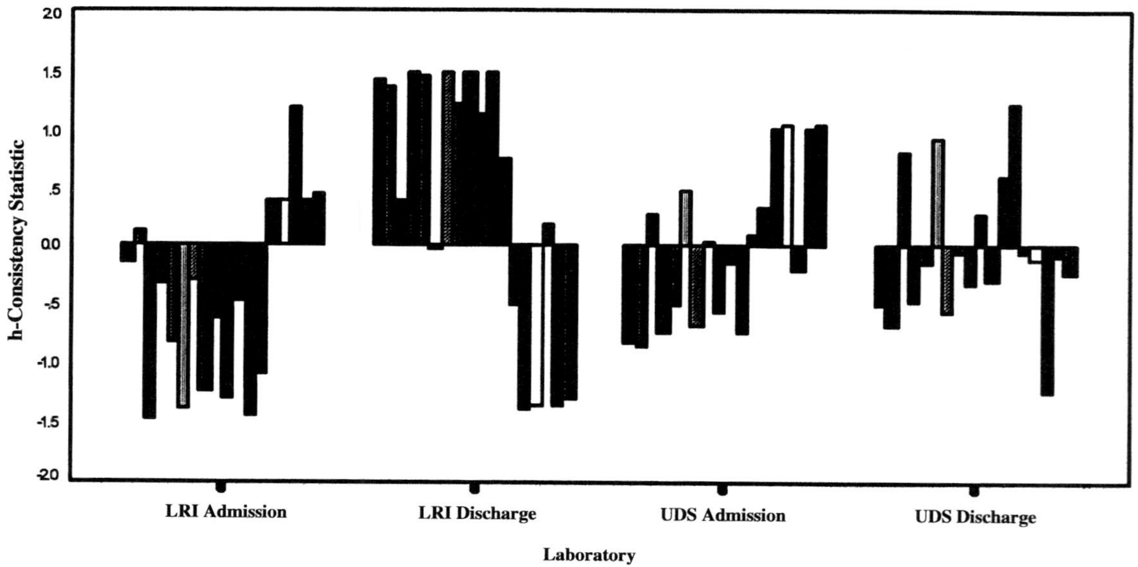

Critical value of h for n of 4 labs at 0.50% significance level = 1.49.

No values are greater than |1.49|.

Each series of FIM items are in entry order, A–R.

FIGURE 8. FIM Calibrations: Items within laboratories.

ASTM and Rasch Measurement

ASTM is a natural partner for Rasch measurement practitioners because of the two groups' shared focus on measurement standards, long histories of success in creating and implementing them, and their common interest in evaluating and improving measurement data quality. There may also be a natural place for Rasch measurement in the activities of the ASTM Committee E-11 on Statistical Methods, especially the Subcommittee E-11.04 on the Development and Evaluation of Test Methods, producer of the standard practice for interlaboratory studies referred to above.[5]

More information is available on the World Wide Web:

- ASTM: http://www.astm.org
- Health Care Informatics subcommittee: http://www.astm.org/commit/e-31.htm.
- ANSI: http://www.ansi.org.
- Electronic patient record and medical informatics standards: http://www.medrecinst.com.

THE "OUTCOMES MEASUREMENT ASSOCIATION"

Given the opportunity offered by an existing ASTM committee's interest in Rasch's scale-free models for measurement, and given that no existing organization of medical outcomes research professionals is prepared to take advantage of it, a new association may be formed soon. This new association would work with the ASTM Committee E31 to set criteria for, conduct, and report instrument calibration studies and round robin interlaboratory reproducibility studies, with the purpose of creating and maintaining scale-free units of measurement for the variables of interest.

The historical interest in Rasch measurement among members of the American Educational Research Association and the National Council on Measurement in Education could be enough to motivate these groups to join with existing or newly created ASTM committees for the purpose of creating and monitoring universally accepted standard units of measurement for variables related to educational structures, processes, and outcomes.

The credibility and adoption of scale-free measurement techniques and standards could depend on the existence of a reputable professional organization that advocates and substantiates the claims made about them. Certainly, to focus research and reporting on the reality of scale-free measurement, and on the viability of metrological standards for outcomes measurement, such an organization is called for. Such an "outcomes measurement association" could be expected to sponsor a journal that would provide informed editorial direction, enlightened peer review, and a professional, credible outlet for scale-free measurement theory and applications in the outcomes research arena.

CONCLUSION

The application of Rasch's scale-free measurement theory involves the discovery and invention of a mathematical law. As different instruments intended to measure the same variables are fit to scale-free measurement models, the extent to which the constructs are stable across instruments and samples will be tested. We could ignore the opportunity for equating these instruments until the stability of the constructs and the equivalence of the measures are so obvious that not putting them into a common metric would be a ridiculous and needless way of overcomplicating communication and understanding. Or we could take the opportunity to equate existing instruments and at the same time begin to design new instruments according to the requirements of scale-free measurement. In short, we can let universal metrics happen to us in their own time, or we can make them happen according to a schedule we devise. Either way, universal metrics for variables measured with tests and rating scales are bound to become standardized.

Every time another instrument's data fit one of Rasch's probabilistic conjoint models, a mathematical law gains the weight of more evidence. Eventually, outcomes measurement will come into its own.

ACKNOWLEDGMENT

The author would like to thank Joseph Biundo, Furqan Siddiqui, Eugene Pezzeck, Robert Mipro, Paul Mayes, Margaret Qayum, Karen Ortenberg, Alejandro Perez, and Ronald Morstead of the Louisiana Rehabilitation Institute and the Physical Medicine and Rehabilitation section of the Louisiana State University Department of Medicine in New Orleans for the use of their data. The author also thanks Robert L. Marier and James H. Diaz for their support of this project.

REFERENCES

1. Altman DG, Bland JM: Measurement in medicine: The analysis of method comparison studies. Statistician 32:307–317, 1983.
2. Andersen EB: Sufficient statistics and latent trait models. Psychometrika 42:69–81, 1977.
3. Andrich D: A rating formulation for ordered response categories. Psychometrika 43:357–374, 1978.
4. Andrich D: Rasch models for measurement. Sage University Paper Series on Quantitative Applications in the Social Sciences vol. series no. 07-068. Beverly Hills, CA, Sage Publications, 1988.
5. ASTM Committee E-11 on Statistical Methods: Standard practice for conducting an interlaboratory study to determine the precision of a test method [E 691-92]. Annual Book of ASTM Standards, Philadelphia, ASTM, 1992.
6. Bailar BA: Quality issues in measurement. Int Stat Rev 53:123–129, 1985.
7. Bland JM, Altman DG: Statistical methods for assessing agreement between two methods of clinical measurement. Lancet 1:307–310, 1986.
8. Cella DF, Lloyd SR, Wright BD: Cross-cultural instrument equating: Current research and future directions. In Spilker B (ed): Quality of Life and Pharmacoeconomics in Clinical Trials. 2nd ed. New York, Lippincott-Raven, 1996, pp 707–715.
9. Fisher WP Jr, Harvey RF, Taylor P, et al: Rehabits: A common language of functional assessment. Arch Phys Med Rehabil 76:113–122, 1995.
10. Fisher WP Jr, Marier RL, Allen SH, et al: Comparing probabilistic calibrations of two health status instruments: The LSU HSI and the HSQ 2.0 [Measurement Research Reports]. New Orleans, Louisiana State University, Louisiana State University Medical Center Department of Public Health and Preventive Medicine, 1995.
11. Fisher WP Jr, Marier RL, Allen SH, et al: Equating the LSU HSI and the SF-36 with a probabilistic measurement model [Measurement Research Reports]. New Orleans, Louisiana State University, Louisiana State University Medical Center Department of Public Health and Preventive Medicine, 1996.
12. Gonin R, Lloyd SR, Cella DF: Establishing equivalence between scaled measures of quality of life. Qual Life Res 20–26, 1996.
13. Haley SM, McHorney CA, Ware JE Jr: Evaluation of the MOS SF-36 physical functioning scale (PF-10). I: Unidimensionality and reproducibility of the Rasch item scale. J Clin Epidemiol 47:671–684, 1994.
14. Hedges LV: How hard is hard science, how soft is soft science? The empirical cumulativeness of research. J Am Psychol Assoc 42:443–445, 1987.
15. Heinemann AW, Linacre JM, Wright BD, et al: Relationships between impairment and physical disability as measured by the Functional Independence Measure. Arch Phys Med Rehabil 74:566–573, 1993.
16. Heinemann A, Segal M, Schall RR, Wright BD: Extending the range of the Functional Independence Measure with SF-36 items. In Smith RHR, Wright B (eds): Outcome Measurement in the Health Sciences. Vol 1. First International Outcome Measurement Conference, Chicago, MESA Press, 1996.
17. Hunter JS: The national system of scientific measurement. Science 210:869–874, 1980.
18. Kilgore KM, Fisher WP Jr, Harvey RF, Silverstein B: Diagnosis-based differences in Rasch calibrations of functional assessment scales [abstract]. Arch Phys Med Rehabil 74:1254, 1993.
19. Linacre JM, Heinemann AW, Wright BD, et al: The structure and stability of the Functional Independence Measure. Arch Phys Med Rehabil 75:127–132, 1994.

20. Mandel J: Interlaboratory testing. ASTM Standardization News 6:11–12, December 1978.
21. Mandel J: The analysis of interlaboratory test data. ASTM Standardization News 5:17–20, 56, March 1977.
22. Masters GN: A Rasch model for partial credit scoring. Psychometrika 47:149–174, 1982.
23. Masters GN: Common-person equating with the Rasch model. Appl Psychol Measure 9:73–82, 1985.
24. Masters G, Wright BD: The essential process in a family of measurement models. Psychometrika 49:529–544, 1984.
25. Mayes P, Perez A, Mipro RC Jr, Fisher WP Jr: Comparison of Functional Independence Measure data from the Uniform Data System and Louisiana Rehabilitation Institute [abstract]. New Orleans, Louisiana State University, Louisiana State University Department of Medicine, Section of Physical Medicine & Rehabilitation, Louisiana State University School of Medicine, 1996.
26. O'Connell J: Metrology: The creation of universality by the circulation of particulars. Social Stud Sci 23:129–173, 1993.
27. Qayum M, Ortenberg K, Morstead R, et al: Measuring functional status in rehabilitation: Louisiana Rehabilitation Institute vs. Uniform Data System [abstract]. New Orleans, Louisiana State University, Louisiana State University Department of Medicine, Section of Physical Medicine & Rehabilitation, Louisiana State University School of Medicine, 1996.
28. Rasch G: On general laws and the meaning of measurement in pathology. In Proceedings of the Fourth Berkeley Symposium on Mathematical Statistics and Probability. Berkeley, CA, University of California Press, 1961, pp 321–333.
29. Rasch G: Probabilistic Models for Some Intelligence and Attainment Tests [reprint]. Copenhagen, Danmarks Paedogogiske Institut, 1980.
30. Schaffer S: Late Victorian metrology and its instrumentation: A manufactory of Ohms. In Bud R, Cozzens SE (eds): Invisible Connections: Instruments, Institutions, and Science. Bellingham, WA, SPIE Optical Engineering Press, 1992, pp 23–56.
31. Velozo CA, Magalhaes LC, Pan A, Leiter P: Functional scale discrimination at admission and discharge: Rasch analysis of the Level of Rehabilitation Scale-III. Arch Phys Med Rehabil 76:705–712, 1995.
32. Wernimont G: Careful intralaboratory study must come first. ASTM Standardization News 6:11–12, December 1978.
33. Wernimont G: Ruggedness evaluation of test procedures. ASTM Standardization News 5:13–16, March 1977.
34. Widmalm S: On exactitude, a review of the The Values of Precision by M. Norton Wise. Science, May 12, 1995.
35. Wright BD: Despair and hope for educational measurement. Contemp Educ Rev 3:281–288, 1984.
36. Wright BD: Sample-free test calibration and person measurement. In Proceedings of the 1967 Invitational Conference on Testing Problems. Princeton, NJ, Educational Testing Service, 1968, pp 85–101.
37. Wright BD: Solving measurement problems with the Rasch model. J Educ Measure 14:97–116, 1977.
38. Wright BD, Linacre JM, Heinemann AW: Measuring functional status in rehabilitation. Phys Med Rehabil Clin North Am 4:475–491, 1993.
39. Wright BD, Masters GN: Rating Scale Analysis: Rasch Measurement. Chicago, MESA Press, 1982.
40. Zupko RE: British Weights and Measures: A History from Antiquity to the Seventeenth Century. Madison, WI, University of Wisconsin Press, 1977.

A. TENNANT, BA
C. YOUNG, MD

COMA TO COMMUNITY: CONTINUITY IN MEASUREMENT

From the Rheumatology and Rehabilitation Research Unit
University of Leeds
Leeds, England
and
The Walton Centre for Neurology and Neurosurgery
Liverpool, England (CY)

Reprint requests to:
A. Tennant, BA
University of Leeds
Rheumatology and Rehabilitation Research Unit
36 Clarendon Road
Leeds LS2 9NZ
United Kingdom

During the past five years the United Kingdom National Health Service has undergone a number of changes in policy and related priorities for health care, in the way in which the NHS is organized, and in an increased emphasis on contracting for health care where there is clear evidence that such care works. Such an emphasis on evidence-led medicine has resulted in an increased focus on the range and quality of outcome measures used to provide that evidence.

This focus has taken the form of numerous reviews of outcome measures, most of which pay some attention to traditional psychometric properties such as validity, reliability and, more recently, responsiveness.[2,7,19] Only occasionally is mention made of basic measurement properties such as dimensionality or level of scaling, which refers to ordinal or interval scales. With regard to unidimensionality, there has been some confusion over the use of coefficient α (Cronbach's Alpha).[4] Recent work has shown that while it can be used as an indication of the connectedness of items within a scale, it does not confirm unidimensionality.[3] Indeed, it is possible to have two or more dimensions in a large item set that nevertheless give a high α.

Internal consistency using α is thus no guide to whether the items of a scale belong to a single underlying construct. Yet most reviews use this statistic to at least imply unidimensionality. This leads to the prospect that many of the measures in everyday use may be suspect regarding their dimensionality, and thus construct validity and responsiveness may be jeopardized. For example, where items are added together from different constructs, overall change scores may be curtailed because items in one dimension are changing at a different rate than another or, in the worst case, are changing in different directions. With regard to whether a scale is ordinal or interval in its measurement, it is rare to find this matter discussed, even in the original papers presenting validity and reliability findings. Yet such properties are crucial to the analysis of these instruments and the choice of appropriate statistical techniques.

A number of issues follow from these shortcomings in knowledge about instruments. Do they truly measure a single construct? Are they at the interval scale level? Are they responsive to change, and does this responsiveness vary according to the circumstances in which change is being measured? For example, can an instrument be used both in the hospital ward and in follow-up in the community? Determining whether the skills learned and relearned in a hospital rehabilitation ward are sustained six months after discharge may be an important factor in understanding the efficacy of competing rehabilitation programs. In this way, a measure to cover the transition from the hospital to the community becomes an essential prerequisite to evidence-led medicine. Again, little evidence is available to inform potential users about which instrument will accomplish this task. In particular, standard reporting of floor and ceiling effects for measures used on patients in different settings is far from an accepted practice. Yet ceiling effects will invariably curtail responsiveness and understate the true magnitude of change.

This chapter examines these issues with respect to patients entering a regional neurosciences facility in the United Kingdom. It examines two instruments that taken separately could not be expected to address the transition from hospital to community, although one instrument is usually used in that context. It also shows how a particular mathematical model offers the potential for harnessing the power of both instruments into a common scale.

METHODS

Patients and Setting

This article considers a subset of 259 patients taken from a larger outcome study of consecutive patients admitted to the Walton Center for Neurology and Neurosurgery in Liverpool, England. Patients in the subset were defined as those able to complete by themselves the Medical Outcomes Study Short-Form Health Survey (SF36)[21] following their admission to the hospital (applied retrospectively to the period immediately prior to admission), who had a Barthel Index[13] scored at the same time, *and* who returned a postal follow-up SF36 6 months later with a valid physical function scale. Patients were also telephoned at 6 months and administered the Barthel Index. This subset is in no way intended to be representative of the total throughput of patients and is drawn solely for the purpose of comparing the responses on both instruments at different time points.

The 259 patients had a mean age of 52.4 years (median 53.7), and the single largest diagnostic category was multiple sclerosis (16%). The severity of disease is best indicated by the fact that only 21% of the 259 patients were employed at the time of admission to the hospital.

Instruments

The Barthel Index is the most widely used outcome measure in the United Kingdom for patients undergoing rehabilitation for neurologic disorders.[8,20]

Developed to indicate the extent of nursing care required by patients in institutions, it is essentially a measure of physical disability and associated dependency in self-care. It has nevertheless been used as a ubiquitous measure of activities of daily living (ADL), both in the management of individual patients (for example, to determine when to discharge home) and, at the aggregate level, to show the efficacy of various rehabilitation programs.[9,10,16] Wade recently argued that it was "probably the most widely used and best standard measure of ADL."[19]

The Barthel Index has ten items. In the version we use, each item is scored from 0 (unable to perform the task) to a variable range of points, scoring 5, 10 or 15 to reflect independence or the intervals on the way to independence. These differential weights—for example, independence on chair/bed transfer scores 15, but independence in bathing scores only 5—reflect the original objective of identifying nursing dependency.

The MOS Short Form Health Survey (SF36) also has a 10-item scale of physical disability, called physical function.[21] Each item is scored 1–3, with 1 reflecting most difficulty with the task and 3 representing no difficulty. The sum of the items are transformed into a 0–100 scale in which 100 reflects fully functioning. One item, *climbing a flight of stairs*, can also be found on the Barthel Index. Another item, *dressing and bathing*, is found on the Barthel as two separate items. Despite this overlap between SF36 and the Barthel Index, the index also has continence and transfer items while the SF36 has items related to walking different distances and "moderate" and "vigorous" activities. It therefore appears that the combined items, both linked to an underlying construct of physical disability, measure a wide range of ability and certainly a range sufficient to cover the transition from hospital to community.

The Rasch Model

The Rasch model[15] formalizes desirable characteristics of measurement. Fitting data to the Rasch model allows us to draw inferences that the observations we have made enjoy desirable characteristics such as unidimensionality.[11] Also, where data fit the model, an interval level measure is produced that can be compared with the raw score. This allows a determination of whether the raw score is at the ordinal or interval level.

In practice there is a "family" of Rasch models, including those for dichotomous data, rating scales, and partial credit models.[1,14] Using BIGSTEPS, a Rasch analysis computer program,[23] data are applied to the model. The analysis calibrates both the ability of patients to achieve independence (or steps on the way to independence) on a given item and the degree of difficulty of the items. Where the item is scored as, for example, 1-2-3, the analysis deconstructs each item into its component steps (from 0 to 1; 1 to 2; 2 to 3) and examines how successful people are in taking those steps. This gives an estimate of item difficulty and is then used to make a first estimate of "person ability." In practice, an iterative procedure refines these estimates until there is no further significant improvement in their accuracy.

The Rasch analysis then seeks to combine the person ability and the item difficulty by their difference. This difference must govern the probability of what is supposed to happen when a person of a given ability uses that ability against a given task.[24] Results of the Rasch transformation are reported in logits—the distance along the line of the variable that increases the odds of observing the event (i.e., taking a "step" on an item) by a factor of 2.718. The relationship between person ability and item difficulty can be best understood by the fact that a person with a logit score of

1.0 will have a 0.5 probability of "passing" an item (or step on an item) with a difficulty level of 1.0 logit.

To benefit from fitting data to the Rasch model, it is necessary to determine how well the data fit the model. The fit of the data to the model is expressed by the mean square information-weighted statistic (INFIT), which, if between +0.7 and +1.3, indicates adequate fit of the data to the model. Item INFIT statistics provide information about the responses given to items around the same difficulty level as the person's ability. Conversely, the outlier-sensitive statistic (OUTFIT) says something about items that are at the opposite difficulty level from the person's ability (adequate range +0.7 to +1.3). INFIT and OUTFIT, taken together, allow one to construct a detailed picture of the working of items within a scale. Lack of fit can indicate multidimensionality, poorly constructed or understood items or, when a scale score is assigned by a rater (as with the Barthel Index used on the hospital ward), lack of reliability in assignment.

RESULTS

Dimensionality

Examination of the Barthel Index (admission) item step difficulty showed a range of 4 logits across the first step of the ten items in the scale. As a result, the data were fitted to the partial credit model, the results of which are given in Table 1. The overall fit of the model is adequate, although a few items cause concern. Some patients, who are otherwise quite able, report incontinence of bladder despite the relative ease of achieving independence on this item for most people. Some with higher levels of ability also report difficulty with feeding or with bowel continence.

Fit of data from the SF36 physical function scale is shown in Table 2; the data are from the follow-up at 6 months and fitted to the partial credit model. Overall fit is adequate, but the item "bathing and dressing" shows considerable misfit, both for the least able patients (INFIT) and the most able patients (OUTFIT). Thus, the least able patients report no difficulty and the most able patients difficulty with this item.

TABLE 1. Fit of Barthel Index Items (Admission) to the Rasch Model

Item	Logit Measure	Error	INFIT		OUTFIT	
			MNSQ	STD	MNSQ	STD
Bathing	2.41	.18	0.85	–1.7	0.61	–1.8
Stairs	2.03	.12	0.73	–2.9	0.60	–2.5
Ambulation	1.40	.09	1.05	0.5	0.98	–0.1
Toilet	–0.03	.11	0.70	–3.7	0.57	–3.4
Dressing	–0.20	.12	1.05	0.5	1.01	0.1
Transfer	–0.23	.09	.75	–2.5	0.68	–1.9
Washing hands, etc.	–1.07	.18	0.85	–1.7	0.81	–0.8
Bladder	–1.10	.12	1.50	3.7	3.29	–4.0
Feeding	–1.21	.13	1.31	2.8	1.87	–3.5
Bowel	–1.99	.16	1.12	0.7	1.86	1.3
Mean			0.99	-0.4	1.23	–0.2
SD			.25	2.3	0.83	2.3

Fit based on 244 persons with nonminimum/maximum score

TABLE 2. Fit of SF36 Physical Function Items (At Follow-up) to the Rasch Model

Item (Subscale)	Logit Measure	Error	INFIT		OUTFIT	
			MNSQ	STD	MNSQ	STD
Vigorous activities	3.35	.23	1.07	0.4	0.71	–0.3
Climb several stairs	1.24	.18	0.84	–1.1	0.61	–1.1
Walk over mile	1.22	.18	0.90	–0.7	0.54	–1.0
Moderate activities	0.22	.17	1.06	0.5	1.04	0.2
Lifting groceries	0.08	.17	0.94	–0.5	0.82	–0.8
Bending/kneeling	–0.11	.17	1.18	1.7	1.20	1.1
Walk half mile	–0.22	.17	0.80	–1.8	0.65	–1.8
Climb one flight	–1.55	.17	0.69	–3.4	0.61	–3.1
Walk 100 yards	–1.68	.16	0.86	–1.3	0.81	–0.9
Bathing and dressing	–2.55	.18	1.52	4.2	1.77	3.7
Mean			0.99	–0.2	0.88	–0.4
SD			.23	2.0	.36	1.6

Fit based on 177 persons with nonminimum/maximum score

It is possible that the "bathing and dressing" item has caused problems because the activities are different with respect to the skills required. The activities are also different in their degree of difficulty, with bathing being the most difficult item on the Barthel Index; in contrast, dressing, which is much closer to average item difficulty, is 2.6 logits easier than bathing. Multiple indicators in a single item, as presented in the physical function scale, render the item opaque with respect to how it works, particularly when the indicators have different levels of difficulty. We cannot tell what the patient is responding to. In this respect the item is poor, and we cannot tell whether the opacity rather than a lack of dimensionality causes the misfit. On the whole, however, the physical function scale does appear to offer a single construct of physical disability.

The Barthel Index, on the other hand, has problems with the misfit of the continence items of bladder and bowel. This may indicate multidimensionality and is consistent with previous findings on fit of the Barthel Index to the Rasch model.[17] Furthermore, the item "feeding" needs further examination. Cutting food and spreading butter are different activities that require different skills, which may cause inconsistencies in responses. Alternatively, the item may carry a different degree of difficulty for different diagnostic groups, leading to misfit and undermining the construct validity of the scale.

Level of Scaling

Following fit of the data to the model, it is possible to compare the "person measure" derived from the Rasch analysis with the raw score derived from summing the items. In both scales, the raw scores represent different levels of ability at the margins of the scale than at the center. For the Barthel Index, raw scores below 15 and above 85 represent ability intervals at least 50% greater than those within these parameters. For the physical function scale, raw scores below 25 and above 85 represent ability levels at least 50% greater than those within these parameters. Therefore, raw scores from both instruments should be treated as ordinal data or transformed using fit to the Rasch model.

TABLE 3. Percent of Patients with Minimum (Floor) and Maximum (Ceiling) Scores on the Barthel Index and the SF36 Physical Function Scale, at Admission and Six Months after Discharge

	% Floor	% Ceiling	Mean	Median
Admission				
Barthel Index	4	2	59.9	65.0
SF36	30	4	23.1	10.0
Six months after discharge				
Barthel Index	1	30	76.7	85.0
SF36	26	5	30.7	15.0

Responsiveness

Table 3 shows the proportion of patients at the floor and ceiling of each scale at admission and at 6 months follow-up, together with mean and median scores. While in the hospital, relatively few patients (6%) were performing either at the floor or ceiling of the Barthel Index. As might be expected, this was not so for the physical function scale, with 30% of patients scoring zero. At follow-up, 30% of patients had a maximum score on the Barthel and 26% had a minimum score on the physical function scale. This suggests a very broad range of ability on the physical disability construct, which neither scale could address on its own. The responsiveness to change of the Barthel Index can be expressed by an effect size of 0.64, and that of the physical function scale by an effect size of 0.27.

Cocalibration

To determine whether it would be possible to combine the items from both scales to provide a single measure of physical disability spanning the disability levels encompassed by the transition from hospital to home, Fisher and colleagues set down the requirements for a formal approach to cocalibration of instruments.[6] A prerequisite to cocalibration is that the instruments have already been independently calibrated on large numbers of patients and that their items already exhibit stable and similar scale values. There is probably sufficient published work on the physical function scale to support this requirement,[12] but certainly not on the Barthel Index.[17] However, ongoing work in the United Kingdom on different data sets using the Barthel Index is consistently providing stable and similar scale values. This provides sufficient grounds for an exploratory cocalibration of the two scales, pending further published results.

Table 4 shows the item calibrations at admission for the combined set of items measuring physical disability. The fit of these items to the model suggests a strong underlying construct of physical disability. The connectedness of the items from the two scales is highlighted by the equal logit value for the two bathing items and from the fact that the *bathing and dressing* item from the physical function scale almost perfectly dissects, in logit terms, the values associated with these two separate items in the Barthel Index.

There is some misfit, e.g., the Barthel *ambulation* item. There is also some dependency in the data, e.g., in the physical function item *walking half a mile*. Dependency—conforming to the hierarchical structure of responses more than expected—has been viewed as indicative of the strength of dimensionality.[12] Some high values of OUTFIT indicate more able patients reporting difficulty with the Barthel bladder, transfer, feeding and bowel items. Setting aside bladder and bowel, transfer is essentially a need for help to get from bed to chair and back. Some patients who are unable to walk and require help to transfer from bed to wheelchair

TABLE 4. Cocalibration of Barthel Index Items and SF36 Physical Function Items at Admission

Item	Logit Measure	Error	INFIT		OUTFIT	
			MNSQ	STD	MNSQ	STD
Vigorous activities	2.09	.16	1.21	1.1	0.88	–0.2
Walk over mile	1.54	.13	0.73	–2.0	**0.39**	–1.6
Climb several stairs	1.47	.13	0.66	–3.0	0.76	–0.8
Walk half mile	1.22	.12	0.67	–3.0	**0.34**	–2.2
Bathing	1.14	.17	1.04	0.4	0.80	–1.0
Lifting groceries	1.01	.12	0.86	–1.5	0.81	–1.2
Moderate activities	0.99	.12	0.76	–2.7	0.70	–2.0
Bending/kneeling	0.93	.12	0.66	–4.0	**0.54**	–3.0
Climb one flight	0.78	.11	0.67	–4.0	0.67	–2.4
Stairs	0.75	.11	1.22	2.1	1.00	0.0
Walk 100 yards	0.58	.11	0.73	–3.3	0.79	–1.6
Ambulation	0.20	.08	**1.52**	4.6	**1.67**	1.8
Bathing and dressing	–0.09	.11	0.82	–2.4	0.90	–1.2
Toilet	–1.09	.10	0.96	–0.5	1.32	1.9
Dressing	–1.25	.11	1.21	2.3	**1.61**	4.6
Transfer	–1.26	.08	1.15	1.4	**2.71**	6.1
Bladder	–2.06	.12	1.33	2.6	**2.89**	3.7
Washing hands, etc.	–2.08	.17	0.91	–1.1	0.90	–0.4
Feeding	–2.17	.12	**1.37**	3.3	**2.58**	5.7
Bowel	–2.87	.15	1.09	0.6	**1.64**	1.1
Mean			0.98	–0.5	1.19	0.4
SD			.26	2.6	0.74	2.7

Italicized items are Barthel Index
Fit based on 252 persons with nonminimum/maximum score

may otherwise by quite able, thus causing the transfer item to show inconsistency in its hierarchical pattern between different groups of patients.

Following this initial cocalibration, item difficulties were compared across time. When the stability of items had been confirmed, item difficulties were calculated on data from both time points, and person scores at each time point were calculated based on anchored items. Figure 1 shows the comparison of the raw score change from the Barthel Index with that of the new cocalibrated measure, the latter reset to a range of 0 to 100, and, thus, a possible change score from –100 to 100. Most patients had improved, as indicated by the positive change scores. However, each raw score change on the Barthel masked a substantive change on the underlying measure. For example, those who appeared not to have changed on the Barthel Index had a range of –15 to +25 on the new measure. Those who had gained 15 points on the Barthel had a range of –10 to 55 points on the measure.

DISCUSSION

The lack of adequate measures to address the issue of transition from hospital to community is a major barrier to the promotion of evidence-led medicine and to the

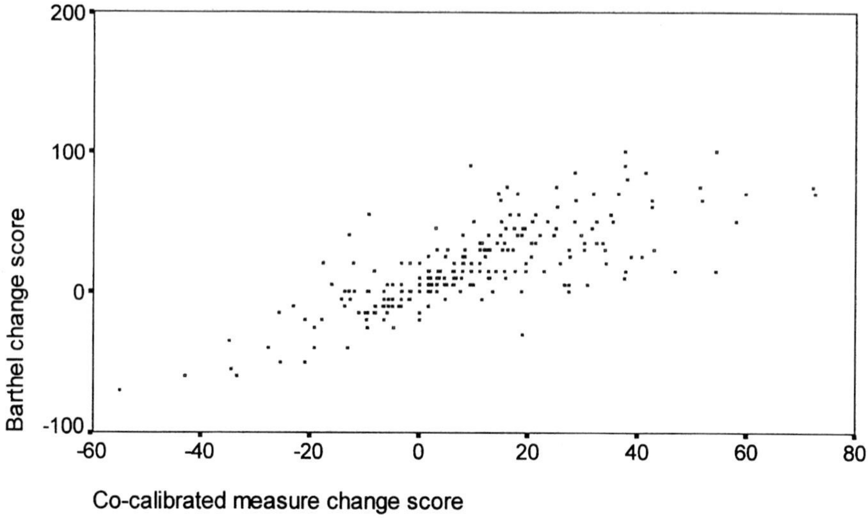

FIGURE 1. Comparison of Barthel Index and cocalibrated measure change scores.

evaluation of competing rehabilitation programs. Using items from different instruments provides the opportunity to address these crucial measurement issues. While the Rasch model offers a powerful diagnostic tool to undertake this task, a prerequisite to cocalibration (or to understanding the construct validity of any instrument) is a clear understanding of the conceptual basis of measurement. Which construct is being measured, and which items tap the construct? In 1980 the World Health Organization published its International Classification of Impairments, Disabilities and Handicaps (ICIDH),[22] which provides a conceptual framework for outcome associated with disease or injury. The ICIDH describes itself as a manual of classification relating to the consequences of disease and as such helps us to view the disease process in a way that would be relevant to everyone involved with care. The conceptual model is clear and simple. Disease may give rise to impairment, which is defined as "any loss or abnormality of psychological, physiological, or anatomical structure or function." This may give rise to disability, defined as "any restriction or lack of ability to perform an activity in the manner or within the range considered normal for a human being." By interacting with the physical and social environment, impairments—directly or through disability—can lead to handicap, defined as a "disadvantage for the given individual . . . that limits or prevents the fulfillment of a role that is normal."

The juxtaposition of this powerful conceptual model with the powerful mathematical model provides us with the potential to achieve suitable outcome measures to support the quest for evidence-led medicine. In this way the lack of fit of the continence items in the Barthel Index is shown to be consistent with our understanding, from the conceptual model, that continence is an impairment, operating at a different level (organ) to the remaining items associated with disability (performance). Conceptually there is no reason to suppose that continence items should sustain a hierarchical ordering with the disability items, and this is confirmed by their lack of fit to the Rasch model.

Although the cocalibration undertaken on these data can be considered only exploratory, the results raise important issues about the quality of measurement in rehabilitation medicine. The use of ordinal scales as interval level measures may lead to erroneous conclusions.[18] Where floor and ceiling effects exist, responsiveness may be compromised. However, the effect size for the new measure stood at 0.47—less than that of the Barthel Index on its own and despite the latter's ceiling effect at follow-up. This needs further investigation but does raise concerns about the viability of the effect size when used on ordinal scales—when the formula involves change scores and standard deviations—and whether, for example, ceiling effects inflate effect size by reducing the standard deviation of the scale.

Notwithstanding these issues and despite the deficiencies recognized in existing instruments, techniques such as cocalibration offer the opportunity to extend the shelf life of current instruments and address important issues such as the hospital-community transition. In the future, standardized instruments are likely to become obsolete as the power of item-banking is recognized and put into practice.[5,24] With the strong foundation of the conceptual model to guide item selection and with the strong Rasch model to select the best items and develop unidimensional constructs, a calibrated set of items measuring the same underlying construct may enable a subset of items to truly measure from "coma to community."

REFERENCES

1. Andrich D: Rasch Models for Measurement. Sage University Paper series on Quantitative Applications in the Social Sciences, series 07-068. Beverly Hills, Sage Publications, 1988.
2. Bowling A: Measuring Health. A Review of Quality of Life Measurement Scales. Buckingham, England, Oxford University Press, 1991.
3. Cortina JM: What is coefficient alpha? An examination of theory and applications. J Appl Psychol 78:98–104, 1993.
4. Cronbach LJ: Coefficient alpha and the internal structure of tests. Psychometrika 16:297–334, 1951.
5. Dobby J, Duckworth D: Objective Assessment by Means of Item Banking. Schools Council Examinations Bulletin 40. London, Methuen Educational, 1979.
6. Fisher WP Jr, Wright BD: Introduction to probabilistic conjoint measurement theory and applications. Int J Educ Res 21:559–568, 1994.
7. Fitzpatrick R: The measurement of health status and quality of life in rheumatological disorders. Baillieres Clin Rheumatol 7:297–317, 1993.
8. Geddes JML, Chamberlain MA: Outcome of stroke rehabilitation—observing current practice: A prerequisite for targets and standards. Clin Rehabil 6:253–260, 1992.
9. Granger CV, Albrecht GL, Hamilton BB: Outcome of comprehensive rehabilitation: Measurement by the PULSES Profile and the Barthel Index. Arch Phys Med Rehabil 60:145–151, 1979.
10. Granger CV, Dewis LS, Peters NC, et al: Stroke rehabilitation: Analysis of repeated Barthel Index measures. Arch Phys Med Rehabil 60:14–17, 1979.
11. Gustafsson J-E: Testing the fit of data to the Rasch model. Br J Math Stat Psychol 33:205–233, 1980.
12. Haley SM, McHorney CA, Ware JE: Evaluation of the MOS SF-36 physical functioning scale (PF-10): I. Unidimensionality and reproducibility of the Rasch item scale. J Clin Epidemiol 47:671–684, 1994.
13. Mahoney FI, Barthel DW: Functional evaluation: The Barthel Index. Md State Med J 14:61–65, 1965.
14. Masters GN: A Rasch model for partial credit scoring. Psychometrica 47:149–173, 1982.
15. Rasch G: Probabilistic Models for Some Intelligence and Attainment Tests. Chicago, University of Chicago Press, 1980.
16. Shah S, Cooper B, Maas F: The Barthel Index and ADL evaluation in stroke rehabilitation in Australia, Japan, the UK and the USA. Aust J Occup Ther 39:5–13, 1992.
17. Tennant A, Geddes JLM, Chamberlain MA: The Barthel Index: An ordinal score or interval level measure? Clin Rehabil 10:301–308, 1996.
18. Tennant A, Hillman M, Fear J, et al: Are we making the most of the Stanford Health Assessment Questionnaire? Br J Rheumatol 30:576–578, 1996.
19. Wade DT: Measurement in Neurological Rehabilitation. Oxford, Oxford University Press, 1992.
20. Wade DT, Skilbeck CE, Langton Hewer R, Wood VA: Therapy after stroke: Amounts, determinants and effects. Int Rehabil Med 6:105–110, 1984.

21. Ware JE, Sherbourne CD: The MOS 36-item short-form health survey (SF-36): I. Conceptual framework and item selection. Med Care 30:473–483, 1992.
22. World Health Organization: The International Classification of Impairments, Disabilities and Handicaps. Geneva, WHO, 1980.
23. Wright BD, Linacre JM: A User's Guide to BIGSTEPS. Chicago, MESA Press, 1992.
24. Wright BD, Stone MH: Best Test Design. Chicago, MESA Press, 1979.

MARY E. SEGAL, PHD
ALLEN W. HEINEMANN, PHD
R. RICHARD SCHALL, PHD
BENJAMIN D. WRIGHT, PHD

RASCH ANALYSIS OF A BRIEF PHYSICAL ABILITY SCALE FOR LONG-TERM OUTCOMES OF STROKE

From the Moss Rehabilitation Research Institute
Temple University Medical School
Philadelphia, Pennsylvania (MES)
and
Rehabilitation Institute of Chicago
Northwestern University Medical School
Chicago, Illinois (AWH)
and
Good Shepherd Rehabilitation Hospital
Allentown, Pennsylvania (RRS)
and
University of Chicago
Chicago, Illinois (BDW)

Reprint requests to:
Mary E. Segal, PhD
Moss Rehabilitation Research Institute
213 Korman Building
MossRehab Hospital
1200 W. Tabor Road
Philadelphia, PA 19141

This research was supported by a grant from the Moss Rehabilitation Research Institute, Philadelphia, Pennsylvania.

This chapter reports the development of a new scale, the Physical Ability Stroke Scale (PASS), for measuring long-term physical ability outcomes following stroke. No such well-validated measure exists. Although our data are taken from a sample of community-living former stroke inpatients with relatively intact cognitive abilities, this scale has the potential for wider application in rehabilitation. Rasch analysis,[20] a form of rating scale analysis, was used to select and recode items from two existing measures, the Functional Independence Measure[4] and the SF-36,[16] or Short Form of the measure used in the Medical Outcomes Study by the Rand Corporation.

The need for such a measure is clear. The social and political movement toward cost-effective accountability in rehabilitation, as in health care generally, is growing.[9] In this public discussion, the question of desired outcomes has become central. Clearly, the measurement of rehabilitation outcomes should not cease at the point of patients' discharge from inpatient care but should be tracked systematically to document the longer term effectiveness of treatment. This is particularly important for rehabilitation, because the goal of rehabilitation is "the development of a person to the fullest physical, psychological, social, vocational, avocational, and educational potential consistent with his or her physiological or anatomic impairment and environmental limitations."[2]

Thus, the emphasis on development of potential of the whole person after disability necessitates measuring outcomes after individuals return to the community. In line with this expectation, CARF now mandates such follow-up, but does not dictate the specific evaluation, such as the scales to be used or the follow-up interval after discharge. While others have been concerned about the issue of post-discharge assessment of stroke patients' physical disability, which is one of the primary areas of intervention in medical rehabilitation,[3] state-of-the-art tools have not been used to evaluate these instruments.

A 1994 survey of rehabilitation facilities suggested that when post-discharge data were collected at all, the instrument of choice was the Functional Independence Measure (FIM), sometimes augmented with a few additional items. Although the FIM has serious disadvantages when used in post-discharge or outpatient assessment, its usefulness in assessing status during inpatient rehabilitation is clear.[5,7] The major problem is the low ceiling in post-discharge assessment: Many former patients are independent in most activities at follow-up, resulting in poor discriminability among them. If the only purpose of the follow-up is to document that gains achieved during inpatient stays have been maintained, the FIM is adequate; however, the FIM would likely be inadequate to determine, for example, whether one treatment of service delivery model was more effective over the long term than another.

In health care follow-up, an increasingly frequent choice for an outcome measure is the SF-36. An abbreviated form of the original Medical Outcomes Study questionnaire, this measure contains 36 items that survey eight domains. One of these domains, physical ability, is measured with a 10-item scale. Although the SF-36 has been validated through large-scale efforts for various medical populations,[11,12] its potential usefulness for rehabilitation has not been established.[10]

The purpose of this study was to ascertain the usefulness of the FIM and SF-36 scales for stroke follow-up, both separately and when all 23 items from both scales were combined into a single scale. Rasch analysis was used to select a subset of items that fit well together as a brief measure with good psychometric properties. A sample of former stroke inpatients and their proxy caregivers (relatives or friends) was administered both the 13-item motor dimension of the FIM and the 10-item physical functioning scale of the SF-36.

THE RASCH MODEL

The Rasch model of measurement is a form of item response theory, or latent trait analysis, employing a logistic model. A logit, the model's unit of calibration, is the natural logarithm of the odds that can be calculated for any given probability of a response. The logit for a probability of 0.5 (1:1 odds) is 0; for .010 (.01:1) it is –4.6; and for .990 (99:1) it is + 4.6. Because logit measures are linear, they can be subjected to parametric statistics and change scores can be computed.

In its simplest form, for a test based on dichotomous (e.g., independent/not independent) items, the model estimates the probability of an individual's response to an item based jointly on estimations of the respondent's ability (proportion of items scored independent) and the item's difficulty, or intensity (proportion of respondents who were dependent) as a logit. These logits, with correction factors for the distributions of total test scores for the respondent sample, form the basis of new measures that have the properties of interval scaling. Extensions of the dichotomous model are appropriate for instruments with more than two levels of scaled responses,[19] which is the case for both the seven-level FIM and the three-level SF-36.

An important assumption of the Rasch model is that the combination of an individual item's difficulty together with an individual respondent's ability is sufficient to predict the response to the item. Thus, the model tests the assumption that all items have equal discriminability.* The probability of an independent rating of an item of a specific difficulty should increase as the ability of the person increases, and the probability of a dependent rating by a person of specific ability should decrease as item difficulty decreases. Thus, all items should be located along a single, hierarchical dimension of item difficulty.

In Rasch analysis, poorly fitting items that do not conform to the model can be identified because observed responses depart seriously from the expected responses predicted by the model. Similarly, persons who do not fit well with the other respondents also can be identified, and reasons for their misfit can be instructive about the items' performance. Fit is often reported as a standardized residual between observed and expected scores. High item fit residuals (> 2.0) indicate that the item is ambiguous or not closely related to the overall construct; low fit residuals (< –2.0) indicate unnecessary redundancy or overlapping content. Items' infit residuals refer to the fit of persons whose overall abilities are close to the difficulty of the item; outfit residuals refer to the fit of persons whose overall abilities are far from the difficulty of the item. Infit residuals are usually examined more closely than outfit because items with difficulties close to a person's level of ability yield more information about that person's ability than items that are very discrepant.

Rasch analysis also provides psychometric properties of the entire scale as well as individual items and persons. Most important among these are statistics about the range of abilities covered by the items, or item separation, and the range of abilities reflected in the sample, or person separation. The separation of items (or persons) is the ratio of the average error-free dispersion between items (persons) to the average measurement error of any one item (person), and should be at least 2.0.[19]

An important advantage of Rasch analysis is that the measures in logits are calibrated along an interval-level scale; meaningful change scores can be calculated from one point to another, which is not strictly possible with ordinal-level data.[17] An interval scale also permits multivariate parametric techniques such as multiple regression and analysis of covariance, which have powerful advantages over less sophisticated methods in assessing the effectiveness of treatment once the effects of confounding variables have been removed from outcome scores.

METHOD

Subjects

Subjects were 38 former stroke inpatients at Moss Rehabilitation Hospital in Philadelphia. They participated with their primary caregivers in a follow-up study about 6 months (range 3–10 months) post-stroke. Subjects were identified through computerized discharge data, contacted by telephone, and asked to come to the hospital for an assessment of physical disability, communication, handicap, and life satisfaction. Caregivers lived at home or spent time with the patients every day.

* In certain situations, this may be an assumption that the test developer does not wish to make. For example, in an achievement test for children, a few items that are easy for almost everyone may be deliberately included early in the test, on the basis that perceived success by respondents will motivate them to put forth their best effort. For the physical ability scale discussed here, as well as most other situations in rehabilitation status measurement, however, these considerations do not apply, and the assumptions of the Rasch model are appropriate.

Because an important aspect of the study was an analysis of proxy agreement between patients and caregivers for most of the measures, inclusion criteria were that patients had either no or mild aphasia restricted to loss in verbal fluency and slowness in speech. Similarly, patients with moderately to severely impaired cognitive functioning as assessed by several subscales of the Neurobehavioral Cognitive Status Exam (NCSE)[13] were excluded. Forty pairs were interviewed, and two caregivers did not complete all measures, yielding a sample size of 38 pairs.

Sample characteristics have been described in earlier reports.[15] In brief, the sample was almost evenly split between men and women (45%/55%). Medians for both men's and women's ages were 65 years. Twenty-five (61%) were African Americans; 14 were Caucasians, and one was Asian. Twenty-three (66%) were married, and 25 had not completed high school. The index stroke was identified as the first by 22 (58%) of the patients. Caregivers' median age was 54, and 31 (82%) caregivers were women. Twenty-seven (71%) were married, and 17 (44%) had completed high school. A total of 21 caregivers (55%) were spouses of patients, 10 (26%) were children caring for parents, and others were siblings and friends.

Measures

Functional Independence Measure

The FIM is a composite measure of disability that has two distinct dimensions: a physical and cognitive dimension.[8] While both dimensions were administered to the subjects, the physical dimension was the only one used in this study. It includes 13 items on four subscales:

- Self-care, six items: eating, grooming, bathing, upper body dressing, lower body dressing, and toileting
- Sphincter control, two items: bladder and bowel control
- Mobility, three items: bed-to-chair transfer, bath transfers, and toilet transfers
- Locomotion, two items: ability to walk or use a wheelchair and ability to climb stairs.

Each FIM item is measured on a seven-point scale, ranging from total dependence (1) to total independence (7) in performing that item. Thus, total FIM scores for the physical dimension can range from 13 (for total dependence on all 13 items) to 91 (for total independence on all 13 items). In previous studies, the physical dimension of the FIM has shown good proxy agreement, whether administered by in-person[15] or telephone[14] interview.

SF-36

The SF-36 consists of 36 items on eight scales: health perceptions, physical functioning, role limitations attributed to physical health, role limitations attributed to emotional problems, social functioning, mental health, bodily pain, and energy and fatigue. While all scales were administered to the subjects, the only scale considered here is the physical functioning scale. This scale consists of 10 items: vigorous activities (running, heavy lifting); moderate activities (vacuuming, bowling); lifting/carrying groceries; climbing several flights of stairs; climbing one flight of stairs; bending/kneeling/stooping; walking more than a mile; walking several blocks; walking one block; and bathing/dressing self.

Each item is scored on a scale from limited a lot (1) to not limited at all (3). The scale shows adequate agreement between patients and proxy caregivers.[15]

Procedures

Two research assistants recruited the subjects, who were paid $20 for their participation if they came to the hospital to be interviewed or $10 if they were interviewed at home. Only five pairs were interviewed at home. Both research assistants received two weeks of training, including viewing three FIM training videotapes produced by the Uniform Data System for Medical Rehabilitation, participating in two training sessions with the hospital's head of program evaluation who awards credentials for clinicians who provide ratings to UDS, and simulating interviews with the principal investigators.

The research assistants interviewed the patient and caregiver at the same time in separate private offices or rooms and were counterbalanced across patients and caregivers to avoid systematic effects for a particular interviewer. Order of scale administration was randomly assigned so that there would be no systematic effects of subject fatigue.

The Rasch analysis program BIGSTEPS[17] was used for the analysis. The 38 patient and caregiver proxy scores were treated as 76 respondents. Although patients' physical abilities were not independent, the ratings themselves were obtained independently. Calibration of patient and caregiver records together is required to determine whether the measurement scales are used in the same way by each group of respondents. A major goal of the analysis was to maximize item and person separation. Doing so selects items that assess the widest possible spread of ability, even though the particular sample in the study was relatively homogeneous, i.e., all were stroke survivors without serious cognitive/communicative deficits who lived in the community with a primary caregiver.

RESULTS

FIM Alone

The FIM demonstrated a strong ceiling effect with this sample (Fig. 1). The distribution was skewed, with most ratings clustering at the high end. The mean of the sample on the Rasch-analyzed measure, which should be 0 for a scale with good discriminability between persons, was 1.17 logits. In other words, a person at the mean of the sample had 3:1 odds of doing well on an item of mean difficulty, although odds of 1:1 would be expected if the mean of the scale separated the sample into two groups of equal size.

There were also problems with the FIM in the subjects' interpretations of the seven-level scale. Rasch analysis revealed confusion about the meaning of the first and also the sixth steps. Various strategies for collapsing the FIM steps were evaluated to make the FIM analogous to the SF-36 (three levels) and to improve the fit of the steps. The following combinations were assessed:

- FIM levels 1–3 collapsed to new level 1 (limited a lot); 4–5 to new level 2 (limited a little); and 6-7 to new level 3 (not limited at all).
- FIM levels 1–4 collapsed to new level 1; 5–6 to new level 2; and 7 to new level 3.
- FIM steps 1–3 collapsed to new level 1; 4–6 to new level 2; and 7 to new level 3.

The optimal fit was obtained with the last rescoring strategy. The separation between ratings improved, and the 1–3 scale intervals worked well together. This rescoring did not affect the measure's item difficulty (items were still too easy), and thus the measured range of abilities was narrow. In addition, poor fit was obtained for the rescored bladder and bowel management items.

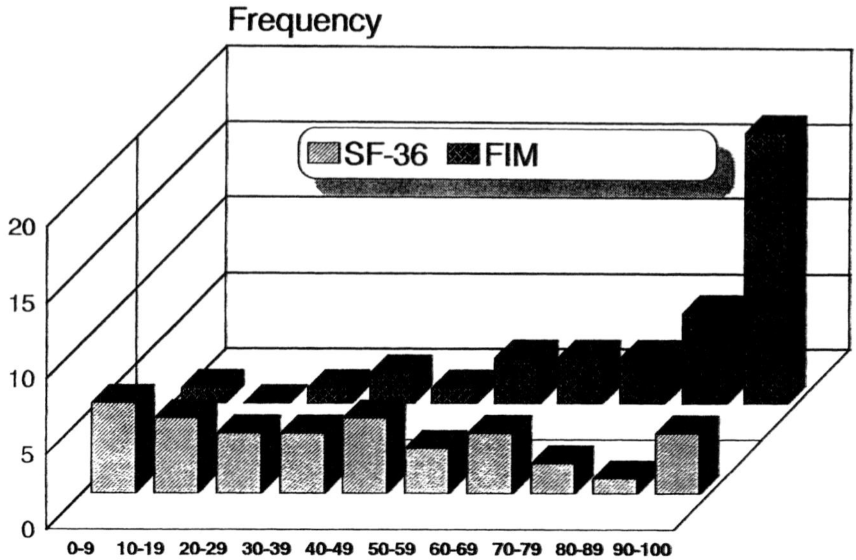

FIGURE 1. Distributions of FIM and SF-36 scores for 38 community-living former stroke inpatients at 6-month follow-up. Ranges for each scales' raw scores have been linearly transformed for purposes of comparison to a scale ranging from 0 (total dependence or limitation) to 100 (lack of dependence or limitation).

SF-36 Alone

The SF-36 physical functioning items showed a strong floor effect (see Fig. 1). The distribution was skewed, with twice as many ratings at the low end as at the high end of the scale. The mean of the Rasch-analyzed sample was –0.59 (probability was about 1:2 that a person at the mean would do well on the an item of average difficulty). In addition, several items fit poorly. The "bend/kneel/stoop" item had an infit standardized residual of 2.3 and outfit of 3.0, indicating considerable noise in measuring physical ability. "Climb several flights of stairs" had an infit standardized residual of –1.9 and an outfit of –1.6, indicating substantial redundancy with other items. There were no overall step problems on the three-level SF-36 items.

Combining the FIM and SF-36 into a Single Scale

The three-level FIM and SF-36 items were analyzed as a single measure. Both the person and item separation statistics were substantially improved, and the mean of the persons measured became 10.16 logits, revealing that items were well targeted on the sample. However, fit statistics showed that a number of items, including those that fit poorly on the individual scales, continued to fit poorly. We deleted the worst fitting items sequentially to select an optimal subset of items that would (1) maximize person and item separation; (2) possess acceptable fit for all items; (3) minimize redundant content with other items; and (4) be as brief as possible, an important advantage for a scale designed for widespread application. For example, the SF-36 "bathe/dress" item, which fit well, was retained and the three FIM items corresponding to this item were deleted. Table 1 gives examples of these analyses.

Table 1 also shows that a solution combining six SF-36 and four FIM items appeared optimal. The mean of this measure was 0.22, close to the goal of 0.00 (odds

TABLE 1. Summary of Rasch Analyses of SF-36 and FIM Item Combinations

Step	No. of Items	Person Separation	Item Separation	Largest Standard Residual: Infit	Largest Standard Residual: Outfit	Items to Delete
1	23	3.69	5.76	2.8	2.3	Bowel, bladder (FIM) Bend, lift (SF-36)
2	19	3.73	6.42	2.7	3.8	Walk several blocks (SF-36)
3	18	3.67	6.58	1.8	3.9	Dress lower body (FIM) Climb > flight (SF-36)
4	10	2.64	8.02	1.0	0.9	Satisfactory solution

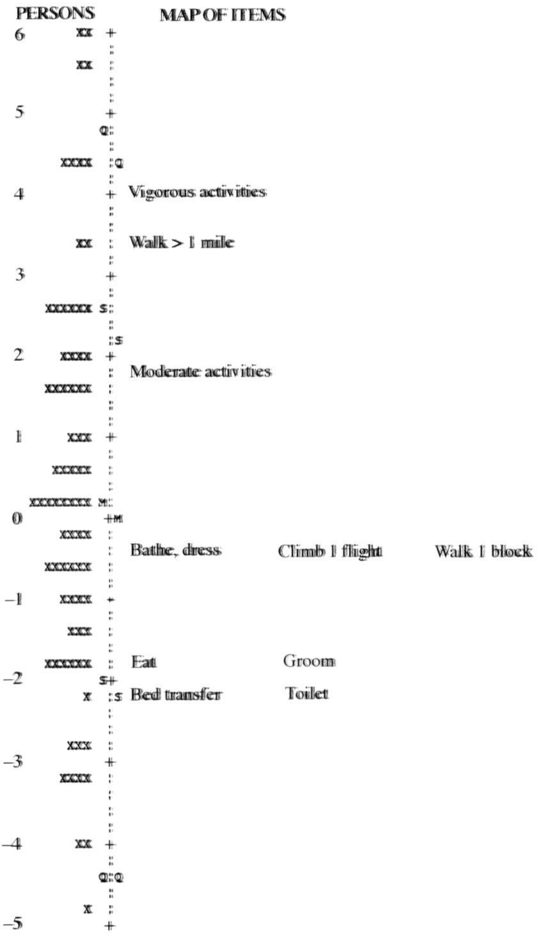

FIGURE 2. Map of caregiver and patient measures (to the left of the vertical axis) and items on the Physical Ability Stroke Scale. Scaled units are logits derived from Rasch analysis of raw scores. M: mean; S: 1 standard deviation from mean; Q: 2 standard deviations from mean.

TABLE 2. Fit Statistics for the Physical Ability Stroke Scale (Items Listed from Most to Least Difficult)

Item	Raw Score*	Measure	Standard Error	Standard Residual Infit	Standard Residual Outfit
Vigorous activities (SF-36)	92	4.05	0.33	–0.2	0.9
Walk > mile (SF-36)	98	3.45	0.30	0.1	–0.5
Moderate activities (SF-36)	121	1.75	0.27	1.0	0.5
Walk 1 block (SF-36)	158	–.37	0.26	1.0	0.1
Climb 1 flight (SF-36)	159	–.42	0.24	–0.4	–0.1
Bathe/dress (SF-36)	160	–.48	0.24	–0.4	–0.5
Eat (FIM)	181	–1.73	0.25	–0.7	–0.1
Groom (FIM)	183	–1.86	0.26	–0.6	–0.7
Bed transfer (FIM)	187	–2.13	0.26	–1.1	–0.2
Toilet self-care (FIM)	189	–2.27	0.28	0.6	–0.5
Mean	153	0.00	0.27	–0.1	–0.1
Standard deviation	35	2.19	0.03	0.7	0.5

* Possible scores range from 74 to 222; 74 persons were measured on the item scale ranging from 1–3. Two persons were eliminated because they had scores of 74, the lowest possible. Rasch analysis always eliminates persons with such scores. Because there was no variation within their responses to the items, they contributed nothing to understanding the discriminability and fit of the items.

that a person of average ability would do well on an average item was 1.2:1). The items in the measure and their Rasch calibrations are shown to the right of the vertical axis in Figure 2. The person measures are shown to the left of the vertical axis.

Analysis of fit of these items suggested that the items formed a unidimensional measure with excellent fit for individual items. Table 2 shows fit statistics for the 10 items.

Analysis of Agreement between Patients and Proxies

Figure 3 plots the average item difficulties as rated by patients along the horizontal axis relative to their average difficulties as rated by caregiver proxies along the vertical axis. The item with greatest disagreement was "vigorous activities," which patients rated as substantially more difficult than did their caregivers. Otherwise, patient and caregiver ratings fell within one logit of each other.

Finally, total Rasch measures of the individual patient and caregivers were plotted against each other in Figure 4. The intraclass correlation calculated on the raw data scores on the new 10-item scale for this sample was 0.77 (confidence interval 0.60–0.87), suggesting overall good agreement between pairs. Using the information in Figure 4, the most discrepant patients and caregivers can be identified and the raw data reexamined for possible reasons.

DISCUSSION

Individual FIM and SF-36 Scales

Rasch analysis helped us develop a brief yet efficient measure of long-term outcomes of stroke rehabilitation. The original FIM motor dimension had a low

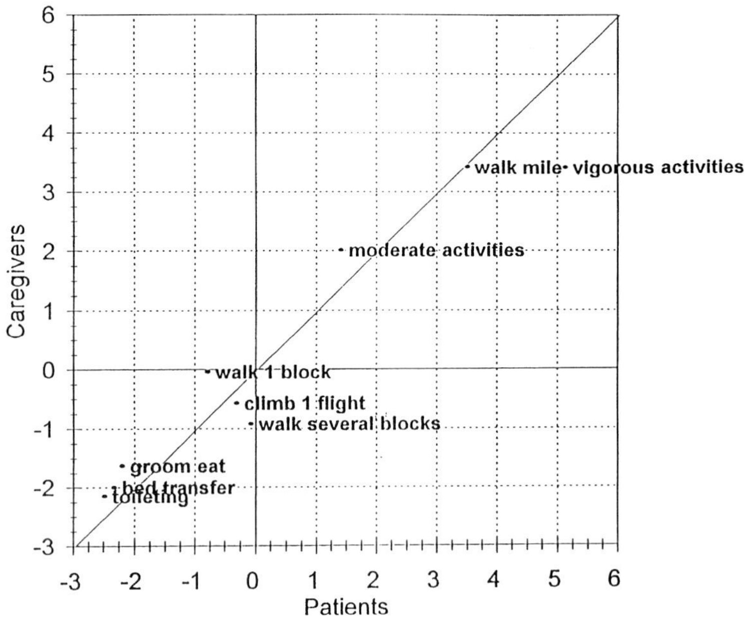

FIGURE 3. Patient and caregiver item calibrations in logits for items on the Physical Ability Stroke Scale.

ceiling, while the SF-36 physical ability had a high floor. In addition, the FIM seven-level scale was not used consistently by respondents. The result was that some people who were expected to do poorly did well and vice versa at two steps. The seven steps appear confusing to respondents for follow-up purposes. Results of this study support a three-level scale for rating FIM physical ability items at follow-up. An optimal solution was three levels, collapsing the original FIM levels 1–3 and 4–6, while keeping 7. This rescoring was used for all subsequent analyses combining SF-36 and FIM items. Validation on a larger, more heterogeneous sample is needed.

In addition, there were problems with specific items on both scales. For the FIM, poor fit was particularly obvious for the bladder and bowel management items on the sphincter control scale. These items also have fit poorly for inpatient samples.[7,8] The two items contain two distinct aspects: (1) usual sphincter management method and (2) frequency of incontinence. Thus, the item is ambiguous and appears to need reworking. An unambiguous separate item should be developed to measure sphincter control at follow-up.

For the SF-36, the "bend/kneel/stoop" item fit poorly, as it did in a large sample of the general population.[6] Because it includes multiple activities, its interpretation is ambiguous. Someone may be limited in bending, for example, but not in kneeling. In general, however, the SF-36 items fit well, although the scale was too difficult for this sample and did not discriminate well.

Combining the FIM and SF-36 into a Single Scale

Combining the two scales into one of 23 items greatly improved the range of ability that was measured. However, because some items still mis-fit, items with

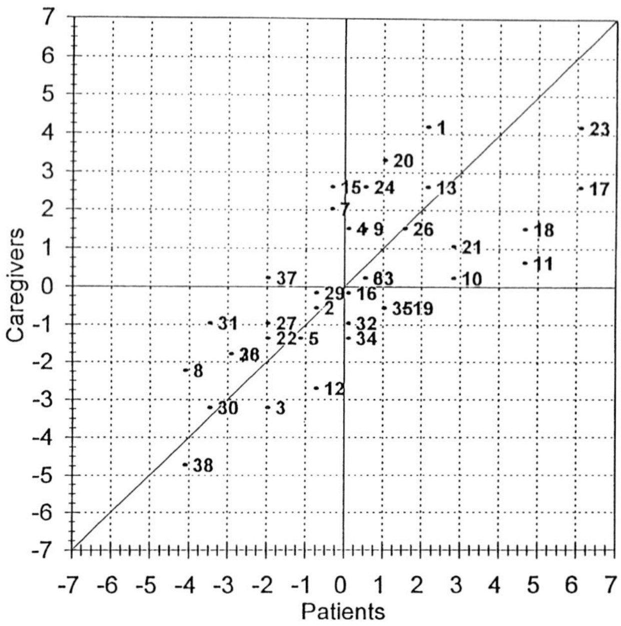

FIGURE 4. Patient/caregiver pairs' total measures in logits on the Physical Ability Stroke Scale.

poor fit and redundant content were deleted sequentially. An optimal solution was reached with 10 items, 6 from the SF-36 and four from the FIM. This subset of items covers all items in the FIM self-care, mobility, and locomotion (except for wheelchair locomotion) subscales. Excluded SF-36 items are "walk several blocks" (a point between "walk 1 block" and "walk more than a mile"); "bend/kneel/stoop"; "climb several flights;" and "lift/carry groceries," which all showed less than optimal fit. These activities are all fairly difficult, and their elimination reduced the prominent skew of the original 10-item SF-36 scale.

Results of a recent study comparing the SF-36 to disease-specific measures for separate respondent samples with compromised upper extremity and lower extremity functions support those reported here.[1] The study showed that the SF-36 discriminated poorly relative to the disease-specific measure for persons with problems of the upper extremities, but not lower extremities; a possible explanation is that the SF-36 physical ability items are mainly concerned with lower extremity functioning.[1] Three of the four FIM items added to the six SF-36 items on the PASS involve upper extremity functioning (eating, grooming, toileting self-care) and so augment the face validity of the PASS for a rehabilitation population. The fact that our sample found these items fairly easy also reduces the skew of the original SF-36 physical function items.

A report of Rasch analysis of the SF-36 physical ability scale using a sample of almost 3,500 respondents suggested that item misfit might have been particularly pronounced for the elderly or for patients with greater disabilities than in the general population[6] and proposed that self-care and mobility might require separation into different scales for this population. The study reported here, however, suggests that these domains can be represented along a single continuum of difficulty, at least for this sample of stroke patients after rehabilitation.

Analysis of Agreement between Patients and Proxies

Agreement between patients and proxies was good, with most item difficulty estimates reasonably close. The poor agreement on the "vigorous activities" item was exacerbated by two misfitting persons whose standardized residuals on this item were large. With this small sample, no further reduction of the sample by eliminating misfitting persons was attempted. However, future larger-scale efforts could analyze person as well as item fit statistics.

Good proxy agreement is essential for any scale to be used for rehabilitation follow-up because of the relatively large numbers of rehabilitation patients with cognitive or communicative impairments that make it impossible for them to respond for themselves. Thus, a good scale should show good proxy agreement so that it can be answered by caregivers who know the patient well; there must be frank acknowledgment that scales without such agreement have limited validity because they necessarily exclude from assessment those with poor cognitive or communicative functioning.

In conclusion, Rasch analysis was useful in identifying a brief, 10-item physical ability scale appropriate for follow-up of this sample of stroke patients. The next step is to validate the PASS on a larger sample of patients, perhaps including those with diagnoses other than stroke, to determine its general applicability for rehabilitation follow-up.

ACKNOWLEDGMENT

The authors thank Virginia Davis, OTR/L, and Pamela Schaffer, OTR/L, for the data collection.

REFERENCES

1. Beaton D, Erdeljan S, Hogg-Johnson S, Bombardier C: Comparison of performance of generic SF-36 and three disease-specific measures of health status in injured workers. Presented at the 1995 International Conference on Health Policy Research, Boston, December 2–3, 1995.
2. DeLisa JA, Martin GM, Currie DM: Rehabilitation medicine: Past, present and future. In DeLisa JA (ed): Rehabilitation Medicine: Principles and Practice. 2nd ed. Philadelphia, J.B. Lippincott, 1993, pp 3–27.
3. Gladman JR, Lincoln NB, Adams SA: Use of the extended ADL scale with stroke patients. Age Ageing 22:419–424, 1993.
4. Granger CV, Hamilton BB, Fiedler RC: Discharge outcome after stroke rehabilitation. Stroke 23:978–982, 1992.
5. Granger CV, Hamilton BB, Linacre JM, et al: Performance profiles of the Functional Independence Measure. Am J Phys Med Rehabil 72:84–98, 1993.
6. Haley SM, McHorney CA, Ware JE: Evaluation of the MOS SF-36 physical functioning scale (PF-10). I: Unidimensionality and reproducibility of the Rasch item scale. J Clin Epidemiol 47:671–684, 1994.
7. Heinemann AW, Linacre JM, Wright BD, et al: Prediction of rehabilitation outcomes with disability measures. Arch Phys Med Rehabil 75:133–143, 1994.
8. Heinemann AW, Linacre JM,Wright BD, et al: Relationships between impairment and physical disability as measured by the Functional Independence Measure. Arch Phys Med Rehabil 74:566–573, 1993.
9. Iezzoni LI: Risk Adjustment for Measuring Health Care Outcomes. Ann Arbor, MI, Health Administration Press, 1994.
10. Keith RA: Functional status and health status. Arch Phys Med Rehabil 85:478–483, 1994.
11. McHorney C, Ware JE, Lu JFR, Sherbourne CD: The MOS 36-item Short-Form Health Survey (SF-36). III: Tests of data quality, scaling assumptions, and reliability across diverse patient groups. Med Care 32:40–66, 1994.
12. McHorney CA, Ware JE, Ruczek AE: The MOS 36-item Short-Form Health Survey (SF-36). II: Psychometric and clinical tests of validity in measuring physical and mental health constructs. Med Care 31:247–263, 1993.

13. Osmon DC, Smet IC, Winegarden B, Gandhavi B: Neurobehavioral cognitive status examination: Its use with unilateral stroke patients in a rehabilitation setting. Arch Phys Med Rehabil 73:414–418, 1992.
14. Segal ME, Gillard M, Schall RR: Telephone and in-person proxy agreement between stroke patients and caregivers for the Functional Independence Measure. Am J Phys Med Rehabil 75:208–212, 1996.
15. Segal ME, Schall RR: Determining functional/health status and its relation to disability in stroke survivors. Stroke 25:2391–2397, 1994.
16. Ware JE, Sherbourne CD: The MOS 36-item Short-Form Health Survey (SF-36). I: Conceptual framework and item selection. Med Care 30:473–483, 1992.
17. Wright BD, Linacre JM: A User's Guide to BIGSTEPS Rasch-Model Computer Program (Version 2.5). Chicago, MESA Press, 1995.
18. Wright BD, Linacre JM: Observations are always ordinal; measurements, however, must be interval. Arch Phys Med Rehabil 70:857–860, 1989.
19. Wright BD, Masters GN: Rating Scale Analysis. Chicago, MESA Press, 1982.
20. Wright BD, Stone MH: Best Test Design. Chicago, MESA Press, 1979.

CHIH-HUNG CHANG, PHD
DAVID CELLA, PHD

EQUATING HEALTH-RELATED QUALITY OF LIFE INSTRUMENTS IN APPLIED ONCOLOGY SETTINGS

From the Department of Psychology
Rush-Presbyterian-St. Luke's Medical Center
Chicago, Illinois

Reprint requests to:
Chih-Hung Chang, PhD
Department of Psychology
Rush-Presbyterian-St. Luke's Medical Center
1653 West Congress Parkway
Chicago, IL 60612

Supported by grant #R01 CA60068 from the National Cancer Institute, Bethesda, Maryland.

Over the past decade, outcome evaluation in oncology trials research has evolved from consideration of measurable tumor response, survival time, and provider-rated toxicity into a broader multidimensional quantification of patient functional status.[4,5,7,11–13,17,21,22,25,30,31] Given the advent of hematopoietic growth factors and improved antiemetic regimens, treatment intensification strategies that increase toxicity are likely to continue. This heightens the importance of evaluating toxicity, patient function, and patient preference for treatment. The subjective, multidimensional construct that is shaped by, but not entirely dependent on, the effects of disease and treatment has come to be called quality of life, or health-related quality of life (QL). QL evaluation differs from classic toxicity evaluation in two important ways: (1) it incorporates more aspects of functioning (e.g., affect and social well-being) than those that have typically been attributed to treatment and (2) it is measured from the patient's perspective.

Many valid instruments are available to measure QL in patients with cancer, but they are seldom used by oncologists. Although quality of their patients' lives is considered to be as important as quantity,[18,29] little attention is paid to available patient-rated QL data.[28] However, this problem is not true of oncologists' use of other QL ratings, such as toxicity, pain, and performance status rating.

A critical question that bears upon the future usefulness of QL data is: Can a common language of QL as an endpoint be developed? This question addresses the possibility of creating a valid and meaningful range of values to represent QL, thus enabling better communication regarding patient status among clinicians and investigators in oncology practice.[16] This has been accomplished with patient activity level (performance status) and pain, where oncologists communicate regularly using numeric scales for performance of the two.[10,14,19,37]

The appeal of universally understood numeric scales lies in their simplicity and usefulness in evaluating responses to treatments. A similar metric for QL realistically could be derived and used among health professionals for group comparisons as well as clinical practice with individual patients. The motivation is therefore to be able to establish some degree of "equivalence" between such scaled measures and thus improve communication between health-care providers. For health providers and policy makers to review data across trials, it will be necessary to have converted scores derived from valid measures.

A number of validated QL measures have emerged and been accepted for use in applied oncology settings. It is therefore unlikely that a single "gold standard" measure will emerge soon. In fact, the diversity of measures that has evolved is potentially valuable in that it enables us to choose an instrument based on specific characteristics of a given disease site, clinical trial, or QL domain of interest. However, without demonstrated comparability and compatibility across the most commonly used measures, communication about QL will be secondary to the practical interests of scale or trial investigators.

The objective of this study was to demonstrate how equivalence of QL across different measures could be established and to develop a standard metric (called Q-score) for five commonly used quality of life measures. The metric will be the derivation of a range of scores that are meaningful across all five quality of life measures included in the study. It is hoped that the creation of a common metric will serve a variety of purposes: (1) to demonstrate the extent to which these commonly used QL instruments are equivalent; (2) to help advance the field of QL by supporting the use of a number of well validated QL measures; (3) to increase communication about QL among physicians and researchers who choose to use different measures for different purposes; and (4) ultimately to contribute to enhanced patient care and quality of life by helping doctors feel more comfortable with QL concepts and their clinical and research value.

METHOD

Participants and Procedures

Because this project was designed to derive universal scaled scores for quality of life evaluation in cancer, maximum patient heterogeneity was desired. Therefore, eligibility criteria were highly inclusive to maximize generalizability. Eligibility criteria include a diagnosis of cancer of all types or HIV, a period of at least 2 months after diagnosis of any particular cancer or HIV infection, a life expectancy of at least 3 months, and sufficient fluency in English to complete forms. Patient populations (oncology and HIV) were screened by chart view and doctor query prior to contact. Eligible patients were then approached by an interviewer, informed about the general objectives of the study, the requirements for participation in the study and about confidentiality issues, and asked to participate. If patients refused participation, the interviewer completed a refusal form. Data were collected from five different performance sites located in hospital settings in different parts of the country.

Mean age of participants was 54.1 years (SD = 14.9), and the mean educational level was 13.8 (SD = 3.0). Most were married and were nonHispanic whites (Table 1).

TABLE 1. Demographic and Clinical Characteristics of the Sample (N = 1,163)

Age	Mean (SD)	54.1 (14.9)
	Range	11–87
Gender	Female	509 (80%)
	Male	651 (56%)
Ethnicity	White	929 (80%)
	Black	176 (15%)
	Asian	9 (1%)
	Other	41 (4%)
Marital Status	Single	226 (19%)
	Married	700 (60%)
	Separated	27 (2%)
	Divorced	106 (9%)
	Widowed	100 (9%)
Years of Education	Mean (SD)	13.8 (3.0)
	Range	4–29
Type of Disease	Breast	185 (16%)
	Colon	115 (10%)
	Head & Neck	119 (10%)
	Lung	130 (11%)
	Lymphoma (no HIV)	143 (12%)
	Prostate	122 (11%)
	Other known cancer	195 (17%)
	Unknown primary	12 (1%)
	HIV, no cancer	96 (8%)
	HIV, and cancer	43 (4%)
ECOG Perfornance Status Rating (Patient Rated)	Normal	323 (28%)
	Some symptoms	296 (26%)
	Confined to bed (< 50% waking day)	379 (33%)
	Confined to bed (> 50% waking day) & bedridden	160 (14%)

Procedures and Measures

Participants in the study provided sociodemographic and treatment information and completed five quality of life instruments: Cancer Rehabilitation Evaluation System–Short Forms (CARES–SF),[15,24] European Organization for Research and Treatment of Cancer Quality of Life Questionnaire–Core (EORTC QLQ–C30),[1] Functional Assessment of Cancer Therapy (FACT) Scales,[6,8,9] the Spitzer's Quality of Life Index (QLI),[27] and the RAND 36-Item Health Survey 1.0 (also known as SF-36).[20,36] Their characteristics are as follows:

CARES-SF

The CARES-SF is a 59-item instrument composed of a list of statements reflecting problems encountered by cancer patients, such as physical changes, psychosocial issues, and problems interacting and communicating with the medical team. It consists of physical, psychosocial, medical interaction, marital, sexual, and miscellaneous subscales. Patients were instructed to answer the questions according to their experiences during the past month. The CARES-SF employs a 5-point Likert scale in which patients are required to circle one number that corresponds to the extent to which they have experienced certain problems. Response choices ranged from 0 (not at all) to 4 (very much). Some sections may not apply to all patients, particularly if they have not received treatment for their cancer. Patients are encouraged to answer all questions that are relevant to their situations, with the understanding that a patient who has not received chemotherapy will not be able to adequately complete the section that relates to effects of chemotherapy.

EORTC QLQ–C30

The EORTC QLQ–C30 is a 30-item instrument consisting of both dichotomous (yes/no) responses and responses that use a 4-point rating scale from "not at all" to "very much." This instrument includes questions related to physical, emotional, and social functioning, along with disease symptoms, financial impact, and global quality of life. Specific questions include issues such as whether patients need assistance with bathing and dressing and the extent to which patients have felt weak. The EORTC QLQ–C30 is composed of functional scales (physical functioning, role functioning, cognitive functioning, emotional functioning, social functioning, and global quality of life) and symptom scales and items (fatigue, nausea and vomiting, pain, dyspnea, sleep disturbance, appetite loss, constipation, diarrhea, and financial impact).

FACT–G

The FACT scales were developed and validated at Rush-Presbyterian-St. Luke's Medical Center in Chicago over the past few years. The general (FACT–G) is a 29-item compilation of symptoms or problems associated with cancer. Patients rate all items using a 5-point rating scale ranging from 0 (not at all) to 4 (very much). The measure yields information about total QL and about the dimensions of physical well-being, social/family well-being, relationship with doctor, emotional well-being, and functional well-being.

SPITZER'S QL-INDEX

Intended by its authors as conceptually equivalent to a neonatal Apgar score, the QLI was originally developed as a 10-point physician rating of five areas of functioning (activity, daily living, health, support, and outlook). Since then, many have used this observer rating scale as a patient-rated scale, with reasonable success.[26] The Spitzer QLI was carefully constructed using expert advisory panels composed of patients and professionals, and it has been subjected to study by at least 28 empirical investigations. In their view, Wood-Dauphinee and Williams[33] concluded that it was a well-validated global measure of HQL. Proxy rating and reliability data for subscales of activity, daily living, and health are more robust than those for support and outlook.[33]

RAND–36

The RAND–36 is a 36-item measure of eight health concepts: physical functioning, limitations in role functioning due to physical health problems, social functioning, body pain, general mental health, limitations in role functioning due to emotional problems, vitality, and general health perceptions. Response choices to questions on this questionnaire vary, but patients are asked to rate the degree to which something is a problem or to indicate whether they have experienced a certain symptom or problem. Some questions should be answered according to patients' present state of health, while other questions should be answered according to experiences during the previous 4 weeks.

Analysis

Rasch rating scale analysis[2,3,35] was conducted. The Rasch rating scale model is an extension of the family of measurement models devised by Danish mathematician

Georg Rasch.[23,32] The rating scale model specifies that the log odds of scoring in two adjacent categories is a function of three additive parameters: person ability, item difficulty, and step difficulty. The log odds is given by:

$$\ln [P_{nij}/P_{ni(j-1)}] = B_n - D_i - F_j,$$

in which P_{nij} is the probability of person n scoring in category j of item i, $P_{ni(j-1)}$ is the probability of person n scoring in category j-1 of item i, B_n is the measure of person n, D_i is the difficulty of item i, and F_j is the step difficulty between categories j-1 and j.

The rating scale model assumes, in the present case, that there is an underlying quality of life dimension. The model has three parameters: B_n, which reflects patients' positions on the QL dimension ("ability"); D_i, reflecting the base position of item i on the QL dimension (item "difficulty"); and the step difficulty parameter F_j, which reflects the relative position of step j of item i to the base position of item i on the QL dimension, with $B_n - D_i - F_j$ reflecting the difference between the patient QL measure, item difficulty, and step difficulty.

A total of 140 items, excluding miscellaneous items of CARES–SF, was jointly calibrated on a logit scale using the BIGSTEPS computer program.[34] A common metric (hierarchy of item difficulty) for these 140 items was created. Patients' QL measures for each instrument were then estimated using anchored item difficulties and step difficulties obtained from the simultaneous calibration. Five separate Rasch analyses were conducted and Rasch statistics obtained.

RESULTS

Cronbach's alpha reliability coefficients for subscales of the five instruments are shown in Table 2. The ranges of the internal consistency coefficients of the subscales are 0.69–0.87, 0.64–0.90, 0.73–0.88, 0.68, 0.77–0.93 for the CARES–SF, EORTC QLQ C–30, FACT, QLI, and RAND–36, respectively. All demonstrate acceptable internal consistency, which is an important prerequisite for establishing equivalence.

Table 3 summarizes the results of Rasch item calibrations for each instrument and combined (common calibration). Person separation statistics indicate that these five QL instruments are moderately comparable, with one exception: QLI has the lowest person separation statistic (0.48). The numbers in parentheses in Table 3 are the person separation statistics that would result if 140 items were created that are just like the items already contained in each instrument. This will allow us to hypothetically compare person separation statistics among instruments if each instrument has the same number of items, which is 140. EORTC and RAND–36 would have higher person separations (6.57 and 6.47, respectively) than the composite (5.55) if 140 items were derived from within each instrument. CARES and FACT would have person separation statistics (5.13 and 5.30, respectively) close to the combined instrument if 140 items were developed for each of these two instruments that were similar to their good items. Item reliabilities are quite similar, except for QLI. RAND–36 has the highest item separation statistic (15.86), followed by the EORTC (12.78) and FACT–G (12.26). Test efficiency (defined as the person separation divided by the square root of number of items) statistics show the EORTC and RAND–36 to possess higher values and CARES and FACT–G to have similar test efficiency.

The five test ogive curves shown in Figure 1 reveal the degree and extent to which each instrument performs compared to each other. Overlapping ogive curves for the CARES and the FACT–G suggest that these instruments perform the most

TABLE 2. Reliability Coefficients of Subscales of Five Instruments

Instrument and Subscale	No. of Items	Cronbach's α
CARES–SF		
Physical	10	0.87
Psychosocial	17	0.86
Medical interaction	4	0.69
Marital	6	0.69
Sexual	3	0.75
EORTC QLQ C–30		
Physical functioning	5	0.70
Role functioning	2	0.90
Cognitive functioning	2	0.64
Emotional functioning	4	0.88
Social functioning	2	0.83
Global quality of life	2	0.89
FACT–G		
Physical well-being	7	0.87
Social/family well-being	7	0.73
Relationship with doctor	2	0.80
Emotional well-being	6	0.76
Functional well-being	7	0.88
QLI		
Activity, daily living, health, support, outlook	5	0.68
RAND–36		
Physical functioning	10	0.93
Role physical	4	0.90
Role emotional	3	0.87
Social functioning	2	0.82
Pain	2	0.88
Mental health	5	0.81
Vitality	4	0.87
General health perception	5	0.77

similarly. The slopes of the CARES and FACT are deeper than those of EORTC, RAND–36, and QLI, particularly in the regions between –1 and 1.5 logits, meaning that these two instruments have better precision in measuring the QL continuum in that range. RAND–36 has a deeper slope (better precision) at the right end of the QL continuum, indicating it has higher precision in measuring patients with better quality

TABLE 3. Summary of Rasch Statistics

	Common	CARES	EORTC	FACT–G	QLI	RAND–36
Number of items	140	40	30	29	5	36
Person separation	5.55	2.74 (5.13)*	3.04 (6.57)	2.41 (5.30)	0.48 (2.54)	3.28 (6.47)
Person reliability	0.97	0.88	0.90	0.85	0.18	0.91
Item separation	13.60	9.62	12.78	12.26	10.72	15.86
Test efficiency	0.47	0.43	0.56	0.45	0.21	0.55

Note. Separation: A measure of the spread of the estimates relative to their precision
Reliability: Rasch equivalent to the KR-20 or Cronbach's Alpha statistic, i.e., the ratio of "true variance" to "observed variance"
* indicates the person separation statistic using 140 items from that instrument
Test efficiency = person separation/√ number of items.

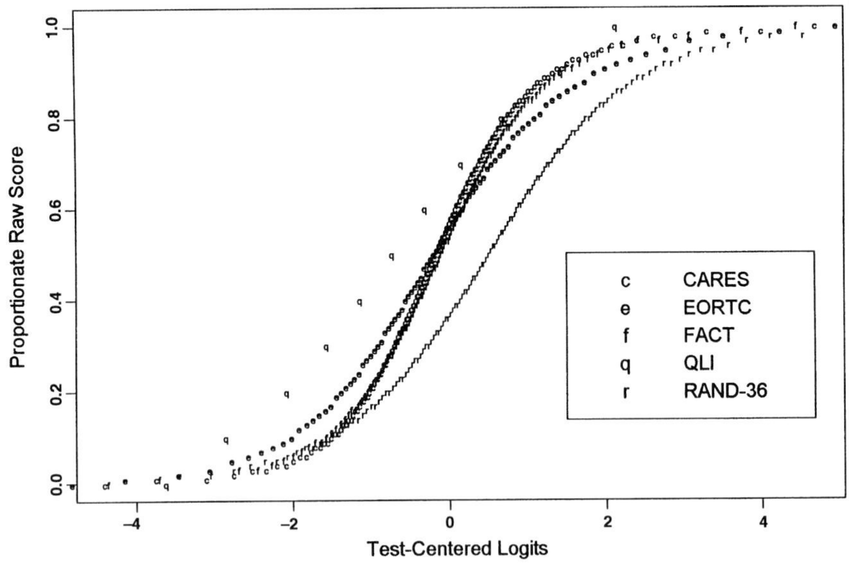

FIGURE 1. Five test ogives.

of life. It is obvious that one instrument has better precision than the others along the QL continuum. These relationships are further illustrated in Figure 2.

The five-test precision graph shown in Figure 2 demonstrates that each instrument possesses a different degree of precision in relation to corresponding test-centered logit, with the RAND–36 performing best (more sensitive) at either extreme of

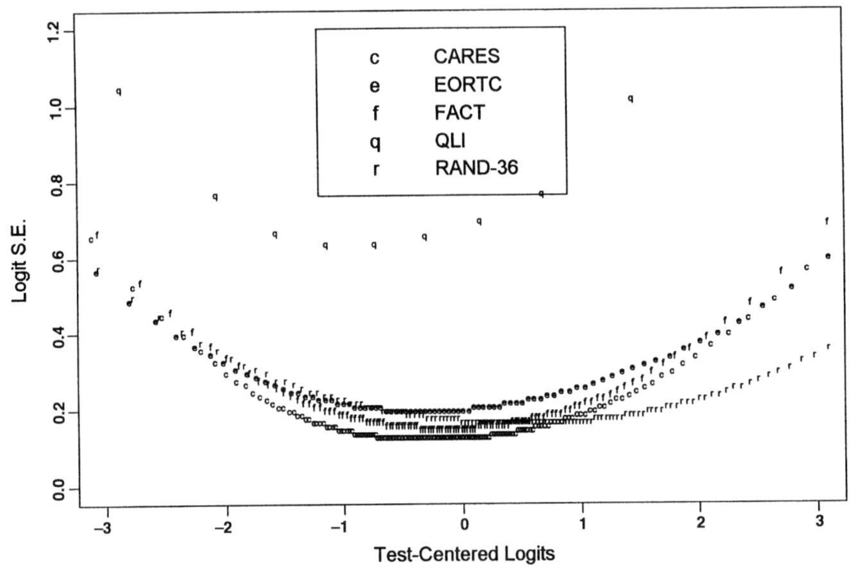

FIGURE 2. Five test precisions.

TABLE 4. Raw Score Equation Table

Equate Measure	CARES	EORTC	FACT	QLI	RAND–36
:	:	:	:	:	:
:	:	:	:	:	:
–0.25	76	72			
–0.24	77		47		77
–0.22	78				
–0.21	79	73	48		78
–0.19	80		49		
–0.18					79
:	:	:	:	:	:
:	:	:	:	:	:
:	:	:	:	:	:
0.14	100			7	
0.16	101	82	63		90
0.17	102				
0.18			64		
0.19	103				91
0.20		83			
:	:	:	:	:	:
:	:	:	:	:	:

the QL continuum (very good or very poor) and the CARES and FACT–G being more sensitive in the middle range.

The equated raw scores shown in Table 4 indicate that the raw score totals can be equated across instruments, using equated measures obtained from Rasch analyses. The sample raw score conversion table is provided as a means of visualizing the relationship between scaled logit and raw scores. It becomes feasible to convert raw scores among instruments obtained from different trials, since correspondence raw score can be established. For instance, if a patient has a score of 79 on CARES–SF, the score can be converted to 73, 48, and 48 in EORTC, FACT, and RAND–36, respectively.

CONCLUSION

Several validated but diverse quality of life measures have become accepted for use in oncology practice. The major problem is that QL measures remain rather diverse in scaling properties, requiring a high degree of sophistication to understand and appropriately interpret data. We have developed a systematic methodology that demonstrates the compatibility of five commonly used measures: CARES–SF, FACT, EORTC QLQ C–30, Spitzer's QL-Index, and RAND–36. Despite differences in questionnaire development, the five instruments measure a similar QL construct. Equated measures enable us to establish correspondence between the raw scores, which can be useful in comparisons among clinical trials and research using different instruments. Although not shown here, conceptually similar subscales and higher-order factors across instruments can be equated using the same equating technique described here.

Another important issue is whether a common language of QL as an endpoint can be developed and whether standard or common scales (i.e., a meaningful range of values to represent QL) for instruments can be derived. Common scales will enable investigators to better communicate about patients' status and enable health providers and policy makers to review data across trials. It is our goal to derive scaled scores ranging from 0 to 100 to form a more accurate and more robust index of overall patient quality of life.

The results suggest that different instruments have their own strengths and weaknesses in measuring QL. The five test ogives demonstrate that each instrument retains different degrees of precision in relation to corresponding test-centered logits. Such findings suggest that test precision could be an important criterion for selecting appropriate QL instruments. Additionally, since individual items from each instrument have been mapped along the QL continuum, it may also be possible to select a mixed set of items according to their precision for targeted patient populations. It would be interesting to further investigate the clinical characteristics of patients, the item difficulty hierarchy, and their relationship along the QL continuum, which will assist researchers in the selection of items to target specific patient populations to yield acceptable precision. Without the application of the already existing measures in research, it will not be possible to judge the benefit of quality of life instruments for specific research contexts. It is hoped that specific studies of the empirical performance of the instruments will yield enough information to assess their use within specific patient populations.

Future national and international collaboration will be necessary to incorporate separate instruments into a universal item bank to allow researchers to develop patient-targeted instruments. Once the item bank is built, it will be feasible to develop computerized adaptive testing (CAT) to administer questionnaires based on patients' responses to quickly estimate their QL and provide timely information for clinical applications. Research along this line should be a logical follow-up.

REFERENCES

1. Aaronson NK, Ahmedzai S, Bergman B, et al: The European Organization for Research and Treatment of Cancer QLQ–C30: A quality-of-life instrument for use in international clinical trials in oncology. J Natl Cancer Inst 85:365–376, 1993.
2. Andrich D: Scaling attitude items constructed and scored in the Likert tradition. Educ Psychol Measure 38:665–680, 1978.
3. Andrich D: A model for contingency tables for having an ordered response classification. Biometrics 35:403–415, 1979.
4. Barofsky I, Sugarbaker PH: Cancer. In Spilker B (ed): Quality of Life Assessment in Clinical Trials. New York, Raven Press, 1990.
5. Cella DF, Cherin EA: Quality of life during and after cancer treatment. Compr Ther 14(5):69–75, 1988.
6. Cella DF, Lee-Rioedan D, Silberman M, et al: Quality of life in advanced cancer: Three new disease-specific measures [abstract #1225]. Proc Am Soc Clin Oncol 8:315, 1989.
7. Cella DF, Tulsky DS: Measuring quality of life today: Methodological aspects. Oncology 4(5):29–38, 1990.
8. Cella DF, Tulsky DS, Bonomi A, et al; The Functional Assessment of Cancer Therapy (FACT) Scales: Incorporating disease-specificity and subjectivity into quality of life (QL) assessment [abstract]. Proc Am Soc Clin Oncol 9:307, 1990.
9. Cella DF, Tulsky DS, Bonomi A, et al: The Functional Assessment of Cancer Therapy (FACT) Scales: Development and validation of the general version. J Clin Oncol 11:570–579, 1993.
10. Daut RL, Cleeland CS, Flanery RC: Development of the Wisconsin brief pain questionnaire to assess pain in cancer and other diseases. Pain 17:197–210, 1983.
11. Donova K, Sanson-Fisher RW, Redman S: Measuring quality of life in cancer patients. J Clin Oncol 7:959–968, 1989.
12. Fayer PM, Jones DR: Measuring and analysis of quality of life in cancer clinical trials: A review. Stat Med 2:429–446, 1983.
13. Fetting JH: Evaluation of quality and quantity of life in breast cancer adjuvant trials. J Clin Oncol 6:1795–1797, 1988.

14. Fishman B, Pasternak S, Wallenstein MS, et al: The Memorial Pain Assessment Card: A valid instrument for the evaluation of cancer pain. Cancer 60:1151–1158, 1987.
15. Ganz PA, Schg CAC, Lee JJ, et al: The CARES: A generic measure of health related quality of life for patients with cancer. Qual Life Res 1:19–29, 1991.
16. Gonin R, Lloyd S, Cella D: Establishing equivalence between scaled measures of quality of life. Qual Life Res 5:20–26, 1966.
17. Gotay CC, Korn EL, McCabe MS, et al: Quality-of-life assessment in cancer treatment protocols: Research issues in protocol development. J Natl Cancer Inst 84:575–579, 1992.
18. Gough IR, Dalgleish LI: What value is given to quality of life assessment by health professionals considering response to palliative chemotherapy for advanced cancer. Cancer 68:220–225, 1991.
19. Karnofsky DA, Burchenal JH: Clinical evaluation of chemotherapeutic agents in cancer. In Macleod CM (ed): Evaluation of the Chemotherapeutic Agents. New York, Columbia University Press, 1949, pp 191–205.
20. McHorney CA, Ware JE, Rogers W, et al: The validity and relative precision of MOS Short- and Long-Form Health Status Scales and Dartmough COOP Charts: Results from the Medical Outcome Study. Med Care 30(5 Suppl):MS253–265, 1992.
21. Moinpour CM, Feigl P, Metch B, et al: Quality of life end points in cancer clinical trials: Review and recommendations. J Natl Cancer Inst 81:485–495, 1989.
22. Osoba D (ed): Effect of Cancer on Quality of Life. Boca Raton, FL, CRC Press, 1991.
23. Rasch G: Probabilistic Models for Some Intelligence and Attainment Tests. Chicago, The University of Chicago Press, 1960/1980.
24. Schag CAC, Ganz P, Heinrich RL: Cancer Rehabilitation Evaluation System—Short Form: A cancer specific rehabilitation and quality of life instrument. Cancer 68:1406–1413, 1991.
25. Skeel RT: Quality of life assessment in cancer clinical trials—It's time to catch up. J Natl Cancer Inst 81:472–473, 1989.
26. Slevin ML, Plant H, Lynch D, et al: Who should measure quality of life, the doctor or the patient? Br J Cancer 57:109, 1988.
27. Spitzer WO, Dobson AJ, Hall J, et al: Measuring the quality of life of cancer patients: A concise QL-Index for use by physicians. J Chronic Dis 34:585–597, 1981.
28. Taylor K, DePetrillo, MacDonald K, et al: Quality of life (QL) information. How do/would oncologists use it? [abstract 1573]. Proc Am Soc Clin Oncol 12: 1993.
29. Taylor K, Skinner H, Feldstein M, et al: Enhancing physician accrual of patients onto Eastern Cooperative Oncology Group (ECOG) trials: Using results from an ECOG survey (EST-C0187) to implement interventions [abstract 1138]. Proc Am Soc Clin Oncol 10: 1991.
30. Tchekmedyian NS, Cella DF (eds): Quality of Life in Current Oncology Practice and Research. Williston Park, NY, Dominus Publishing, 1991.
31. US Department of Health and Human Services, Public Health Service, National Institutes of Health: Quality of Life Assessment in Cancer Clinical Trials: Report to the Workshop on Quality of Life Research in Cancer Clinical Trials. Bethesda, MD, Division of Cancer Prevention and Control, National Cancer Institute, 1990.
32. Ware JE, Sherbourne CD: The MOS 36-Item Short-Form Health Survey (SF-36): I. Conceptual and framework and item selection. Med Care 30:473–483, 1992.
33. Wood-Dauphinee S, William JI: The Spitzer Quality-of Life Index: Its performance as a measure. In Osoba D (ed): Effect of Cancer on Quality of Life. Boca Raton, FL, CRC Press, 1991, pp 169–184.
34. Wright BD, Linacre JM: BIGSTEPS: Rasch Analysis for All Two-Facet Models. Chicago, MESA Press, 1995.
35. Wright BD, Masters GN: Rating Scale Analysis. Chicago, MESA Press, 1982.
36. Wright BD, Stone MH: Best Test Design. Chicago, MESA Press, 1979.
37. Zubrod CG, Schneiderman M, Feri E, et al: Appraisal of methods for the study of chemotherapy of cancer in man: Comparative therapeutic trial and nitrogen mustard and triehylene thiophosphoramide. J Chronic Dis 11:7–33, 1960.

RITA K. BODE, PhD
ALLEN W. HEINEMANN, PhD

AN EXPLORATION OF INTERDISCIPLINARY RATINGS OF FUNCTIONAL ASSESSMENT ITEMS

From the Rehabilitation Services Evaluation Unit
Rehabilitation Institute of Chicago
Chicago, Illinois

Reprint requests to:
Rita K. Bode, PhD
345 East Superior Street
Chicago, IL 60611

Ratings of patients' functional status are usually assumed to be the same regardless of who does the rating. But is that so? Several studies have examined the relationship between ratings of functional status. Many examined rating differences between the patient and another rater and found overall agreement between their ratings.[1,16,18] Some examined rating differences across type of assessment: self-report versus performance,[8,9,14] and a few examined differences in ratings within or across disciplines. Within discipline, one study found good agreement among oncologists rating patients in terms of ambulatory status and need for care.[15] Across disciplines, another study examined rating differences between nurses and occupational therapists and found nurses to be more severe raters of patients on all activities of daily living.[17]

This study examines the ratings of the functional status of patients at admission to and discharge from medical rehabilitation by nurses, occupational therapists, physical therapists, and speech pathologists. A unique feature of the functional assessment data collection at the institution studied is that dual ratings are available for selected items. This overlap made possible an exploration of differences in ratings across disciplines. Previous research found differences in rater severity but did not explore other aspects of rating differences across disciplines. This study examines rater differences across disciplines in the estimation of item difficulty, item misfit, and the use of the rating scale. The latter two aspects are investigated because item fit varies across impairment groups[4] and rating periods[11] and thus might differ across disciplines. A finding of step disorder in the rating scale[10] suggests a need to investigate the use of the rating scale across disciplines.

METHODS

Sample

The sample consisted of 3414 inpatient acute rehabilitation patients admitted for the first time to the institution from 1994 through mid 1996. Ratings at admission and discharge were combined in the calibrations to obtain more stable estimates of functional status and to avoid the skewed distributions of ratings that exist separately by rating period. Four impairment groups composed 70% of the sample: stroke (22%), orthopedic impairments (21%), brain injury (15%), and spinal cord injury (12%); the remaining 30% had a variety of other impairments. The age distribution tended to be negatively skewed; 13% of the patients were younger than 25, 43% were 25–64, and 44% were 65 or older. There were slightly more women (52%) than men (48%). Racial backgrounds included Caucasian (62%), black (27%), Hispanic (6%), and other (5%). The marital status of the patients was essentially equally distributed: 34% were single, 39% were married, and 27% were widowed or divorced. About 90% were admitted from an acute care hospital and 80% were discharged to home.

Instruments

The instrument used in this study was the Functional Independence Measure. The FIM was developed to measure patient disability[2] and has previously been Rasch-calibrated.[4,12] It has been used to measure the functional status of patients with a variety of impairments,[12,19] and its measurement characteristics have been extensively studied.[6,11] The FIM has been used to predict rehabilitation outcomes,[7] study the relationship between functional status and therapeutic intensity,[3] and examine the relationship between disability measures and nursing effort.[5]

The items in the FIM are presented in Table 1 with the overlap of raters and items. For this study, the items were analyzed in four categories: self-care, mobility, communication, and social cognition. Within each of these categories, the numbers of items rated by each discipline included the following: self-care (6 items rated by both nurses and occupational therapists and 2 items rated by nurses only), mobility (6 items rated by both nurses and physical therapists); communication (4 items rated by both nurses and speech/language pathologists); and social cognition (1 item rated by both nurses and psychologists and 2 items rated by nurses only). Since there was overlap on only one social cognition item, no comparisons were made between ratings of nurses and psychologists.

Levels of disability are defined operationally for each FIM item. Nurses (but not necessarily therapists) receive training and are certified on the use of the scale in rating the items. The rating scale ranges from 1 (total dependence or impairment) to 7 (complete independence or no impairment). Self-care and mobility items are rated on the amount of assistance required to perform the task, and communication items are rated on the level of impairment or the amount of assistance required.

Analysis

Item calibrations were obtained using BIGSTEPS version 2.76.[13] The same 7-point rating scale structure was used for all items. Three sets of analyses were

TABLE 1. Overlap of FIM Items and Raters

Items	Rater Disciplines				
Eating	RN	OT			
Grooming	RN	OT			
Bathing	RN	OT			
Upper body dressing	RN	OT			
Lower body dressing	RN	OT			
Toileting	RN	OT			
Bladder management[1]	RN				
Bowel management[1]	RN				
Bed/chair/wheelchair transfer	RN		PT		
Toilet transfer	RN		PT		
Tub transfer	RN		PT		
Wheelchair locomotion[2]	RN		PT		
Walking[2]	RN		PT		
Stair climbing	RN		PT		
Auditory comprehension[3]	RN			SP	
Visual comprehension[3]	RN			SP	
Oral expression[4]	RN			SP	
Written expression[4]	RN			SP	
Social interaction	RN				PSY
Problem solving[1]	RN				
Memory[1]	RN				

[1] The *bladder* and *bowel management*, *problem solving*, and *memory* items are rated only by nurses.
[2] The *locomotion* item is rated in two modalities: wheelchair and walking; raters indicate the modality to which the rating refers along with the rating.
[3] The *comprehension* item is rated by nurses in two modalities: auditory and visual; nurse raters indicate the modality to which the rating refers along with the rating. Speech pathologists rate auditory and visual comprehension separately.
[4] The *expression* item is rated by nurses in two modalities: vocal and nonvocal; nurse raters indicate the modality to which the rating refers along with the rating. Speech pathologists rate oral and written expression separately.
Legend: RN = Nurses; OT = Occupational therapists; PT = Physical therapists; SP = Speech/language pathologists; PSY = Psychologists

conducted on the self-care, mobility, and communication items: the first set consisted of calibrations of nurse ratings on all three sets of items; the second set consisted of occupational therapist, physical therapist, and speech/language pathologist ratings on their respective set of items; and the third consisted of ratings of the other disciplines anchored to the values obtained from the nurse ratings. Anchoring is a means of imposing one set of parameters on the calibrations based on another set of data. The nurse ratings were used as the basis for item/step anchoring since nurses were the most frequent raters and rated the most items; consequently, they were most familiar users of the instrument.

Two methods were used to compare ratings across disciplines: directly and via anchoring. In the first comparison, the item calibrations and fit statistics from the first two analyses were directly compared and differences between them were used as indicators of rating discrepancy across disciplines; in the second comparison, the item displacements from the analysis based on anchored ratings were used as indicators of rating discrepancy across disciplines. Item fit and rating scale use from the calibrations of nurse ratings and unanchored ratings from the other disciplines was examined to compare these other aspect of the ratings.

To compare ratings across disciplines, summary statistics for each set of items and calibrations for individual items were examined. For overall patient functioning on each set of items, the average measures were examined to estimate the effect of raters from different disciplines on the rating of functional status. The person separation indices along with the component error and spread were examined to determine the accuracy of the measures in differentiating patients at various levels of functioning and to identify the source of discrepancies across disciplines. Finally, the variations in item fit statistics were examined to estimate the overall fit of the set of items, and the probability curves for each calibration were examined.

Item calibrations and fit statistics were examined to compare rating severity across disciplines. Differences in item calibrations across disciplines greater than two standard errors were considered significant and used to identify items in which rater severity differed significantly; alternatively, item displacements greater than twice the root mean square error values greater than 1.2 were considered evidence of misfit. The percentage of ratings in each category were compared across disciplines to determine the extent of differences in the use of the rating scale.

RESULTS

Results are presented across disciplines for each set of items in terms of (1) similarity of item calibrations, (2) misfit of items, (3) the use of rating scale, and (4) the effect of differences in rating severity on measures of patient functional status.

Self-Care Items

The calibrations of nurse (RN) ratings and unanchored occupational therapist (OT) ratings are each centered at zero, and the results show the variability in item calibrations to be the same (1.10 for RN and 1.12 for OT ratings) and essentially the same amount of overall fit in both sets of ratings (infit mean square standard deviations: 0.44 for OT and 0.37 for RN ratings). On the individual item level, the item map (Fig. 1) shows the same ordering of items by difficulty level with only slight differences in their positions relative to each other. The eating item was rated as the easiest task to perform by both sets of raters, and the bathing item was rated the most difficult. The item calibrations and fit statistics for each discipline are presented in Table 2 with the item displacement for the anchored OT ratings. These results reveal that nurses are more severe raters of eating, lower body dressing, and bathing while occupational therapists are more severe in rating upper body dressing. Because the sample is large, the standard errors for each calibration are small (0.02); therefore, minor differences in item calibrations across disciplines are statistically but not meaningfully significant. Using a criterion of the item calibration plus and minus two standard errors identifies the cross-discipline ratings for four of the six items to be significantly different even though the largest difference is only 0.13 logits. Using an alternate criterion of item displacement greater than twice the RMSE of the calibration using anchored values identifies all items having discrepant ratings across disciplines. Clearly a more rigorous criterion is needed to identify items with meaningfully discrepant ratings.

Table 2 also contains the fit statistics for each self-care item as rated by both sets of raters. These results show one item, eating, to misfit in both RN (infit mean square = 1.79) and OT (infit mean square = 1.95) ratings with bathing and upper and

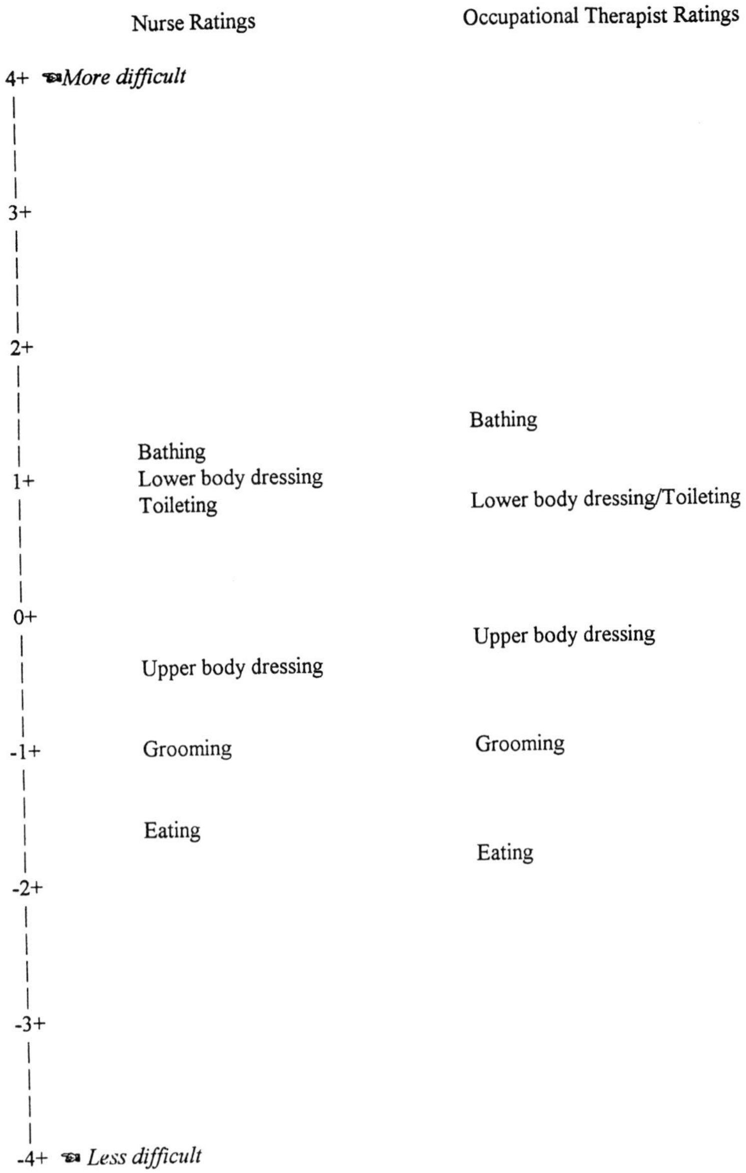

FIGURE 1. FIM Self-care item difficulties by discipline.

lower body dressing ratings tending to overfit the model (infit mean square < .80) for both sets of raters.

Figure 2 presents the probability curves for the RN and OT ratings of the self-care items; these curves are similar and suggest that both set of raters are using the rating scale similarly. Table 3 presents the percent of ratings at each rating scale category for both sets of raters; the results from these items also show similar use of the rating scale across disciplines.

TABLE 2. Item Calibrations by Discipline

Self-Care Items	Nursing		Occupational Therapy		Anchored OT
	Item Calib.	MS Infit	Item Calib.	MS Infit	Item Displacement
Eating	−1.68	1.79*	−1.77	1.98*	−0.24
Grooming	−1.03	0.92	−1.01	1.02	−0.07
Upper body dressing	−0.36	0.73	−0.28	0.76	0.05
Toileting	0.83	1.07	0.86	0.96	0.08
Lower body dressing	1.01	0.80	0.88	0.71	−0.07
Bathing	1.23	0.75	1.32	0.78	0.18
Mobility Items	**Nursing**		**Physical Therapy**		**Anchored PT**
	Item Calib.	MS Infit	Item Calib.	MS Infit	Item Displacement
Wheelchair locomotion	−0.50	1.58*	−0.98	2.29*	−0.85
Bed/chair/WC transfer	−0.37	0.46	−0.66	0.46	−0.57
Toilet transfer	−0.23	0.43	−0.24	0.57	−0.13
Walking	0.26	0.61	0.09	0.97	−0.14
Tub transfer	0.37	0.61	0.53	1.00	0.38
Stair climbing	0.47	3.22*	1.27	1.16	1.34
Communication Items	**Nursing**		**Speech Pathology**		**Anchored SP**
	Item Calib.	MS Infit	Item Calib.	MS Infit	Item Displacement
Oral expression	−0.47	0.98	−0.72	0.77	−0.10
Written expression	−0.37	1.16	1.25	1.61*	2.02
Aduitory comprehension	0.38	0.97	−1.16	0.75	−1.53
Visual comprehension	0.46	0.88	0.63	1.20	0.54

* Misfitting item

Despite severity differences on individual items, average patient measures on the self-care items were essentially the same for nurses and occupational therapists (average measures of 0.92 and 0.90, respectively). While the RMSE is essentially the same (0.64 and 0.63 for RN and OT ratings, respectively), the variability is slightly higher for RN ratings (2.37 compared to 2.22 for OT ratings); as a result, the person separation index is slightly higher for RN ratings (3.57 compared to 3.40 for OT ratings). Thus, although there is no difference in average functional status when rated by nurses or occupational therapists, there is slightly more differentiation across functional levels when rated by nurses due to more spread in the RN ratings.

Figure 3 presents a plot of the patient measures as rated by nurses and occupational therapists for a subset of patients who were rated by both disciplines. Because the sample is large, the control lines are extremely narrow and many cases fall outside the 95% confidence area. (Note: Plots of this type cannot show density of points at each coordinate; the graph points are denser around the best fit line than away from it.) The best fit line does not run parallel to the identity line; RN ratings are higher than OT ratings for patients with high functional levels and lower than OT ratings for patients with low functional levels. The net effect is that RN ratings of patient functional status are higher than OT ratings. (The correlation between measures was 0.89.) This finding was confirmed by a *t*-test conducted on the means of the ratings by nurses and occupational therapists for 4957 ratings (admission and discharge); the average measure from the RN ratings (0.65) is significantly higher

RN Ratings on FIM Self-care Items:

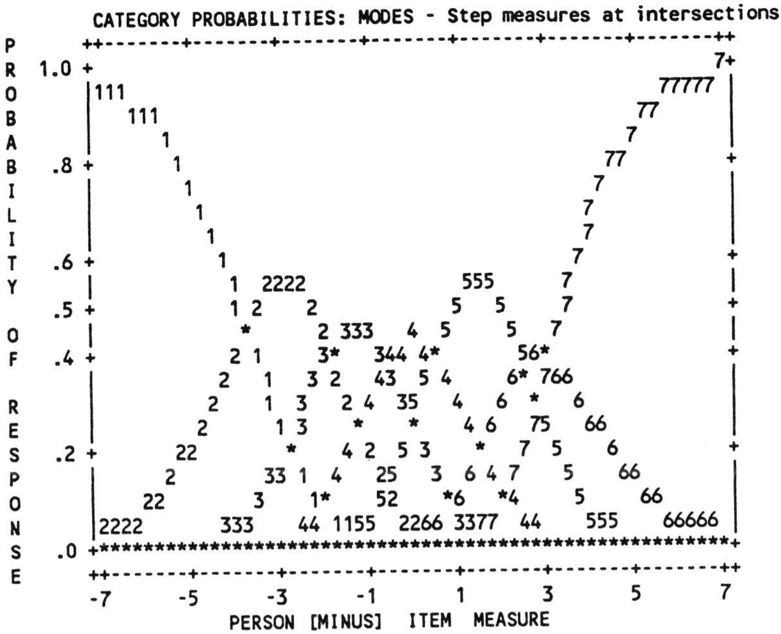

OT Ratings on FIM Self-care Items:

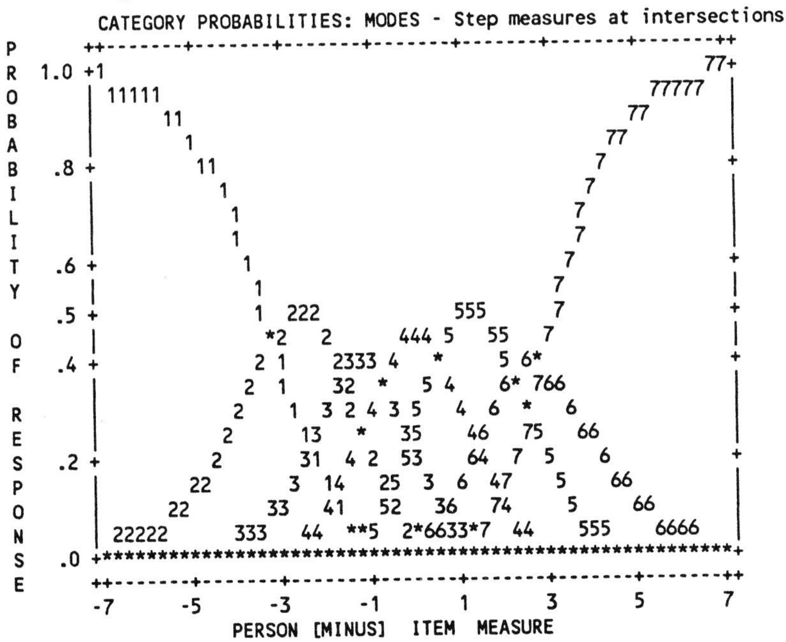

FIGURE 2. Probability curves for nurse and occupational therapist ratings of self-care.

TABLE 3. FIM Rating Scale Use

Rating Scale Category	Self-Care RN	Self-Care OT	Mobility RN	Mobility PT	Communication RN	Communication SP
1	6%	6%	9%	25%	2%	10%
2	10%	9%	12%	4%	12%	24%
3	13%	11%	13%	7%	17%	21%
4	16%	17%	20%	22%	15%	20%
5	23%	22%	23%	19%	22%	18%
6	14%	14%	17%	15%	20%	4%
7	19%	20%	7%	8%	13%	4%

($t = 6.6$, $p < .001$) than that from the OT ratings (0.52). Although this difference is statistically significant, it may not be clinically meaningful.

In summary, it appears that the self-care item difficulty is rated essentially the same by both disciplines; the same item misfits; the rating scale is used similarly; and the average person measures from the individual calibrations show functional status to be the same regardless of rater. However, when ratings are based only on patients show were rated by both disciplines, nurses are slightly less severe raters of self-care than occupational therapists. Differences may be due to the exclusion of

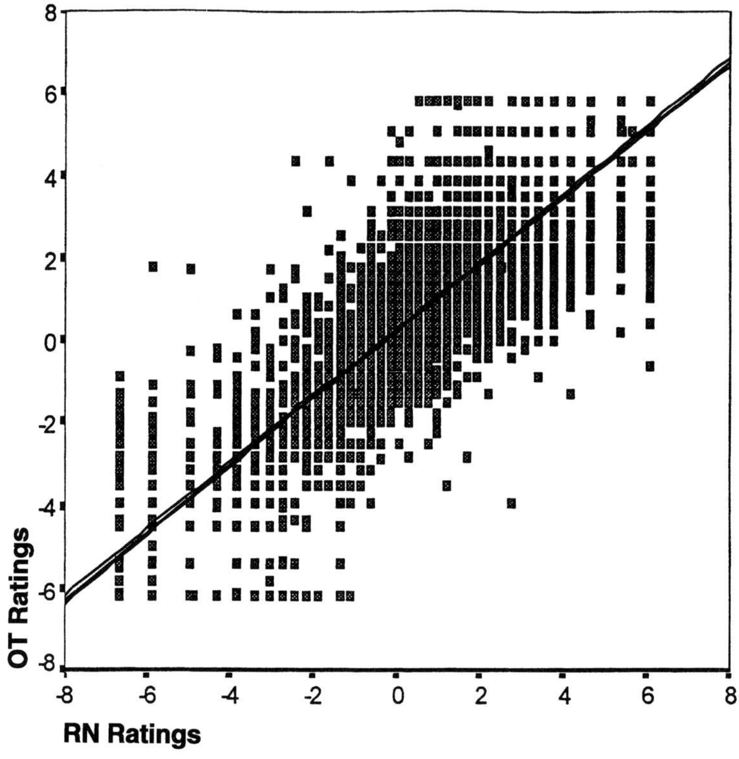

FIGURE 3. Patient measures from nurse and occupational therapist ratings of self-care. Note: Best fit curve +95% confidence intervals.

extreme minimum and maximum measures in the calibrations but their inclusion in the t-test calculations. These conclusions are contrary to the findings of previous research in which nurses were more severe raters of activities of daily living.[17]

Mobility Items

The results of the calibrations of the RN ratings and the unanchored physical therapist (PT) ratings show there is considerably more variability in item calibrations for PT ratings (0.75) than for RN ratings (0.38) and more misfit in the RN than PT ratings (infit mean square standard deviation of 0.98 and 0.60, respectively). On the individual item level, the item map (Fig. 4) shows the same

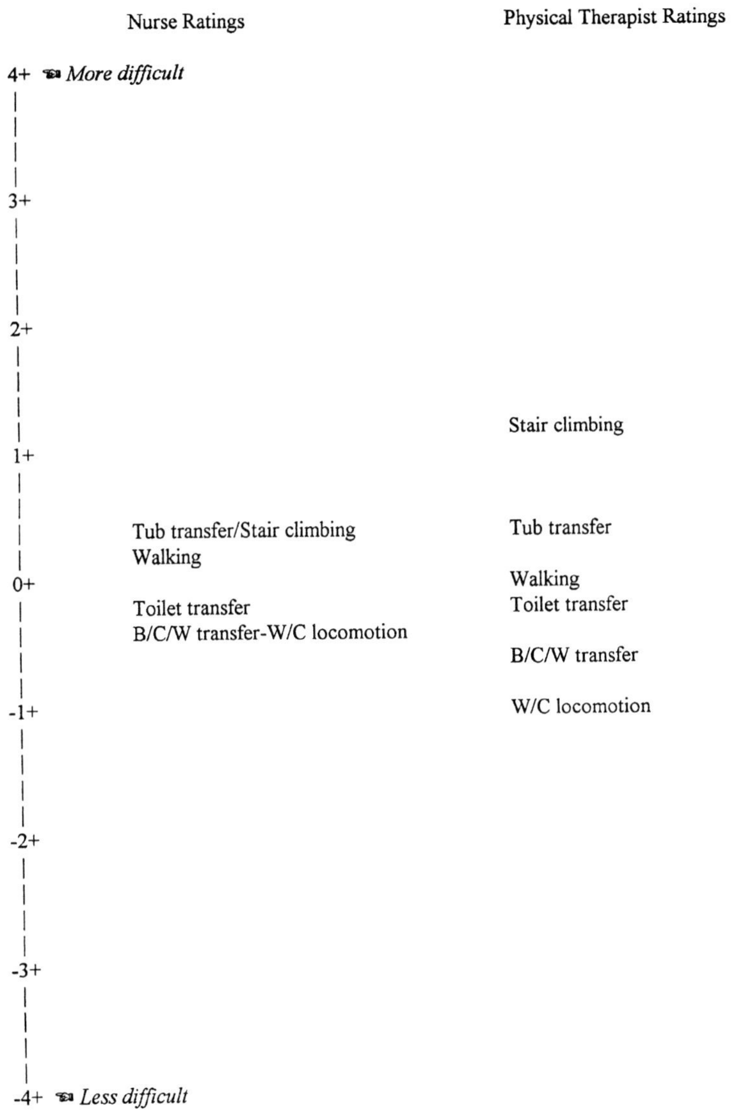

FIGURE 4. Mobility item difficulties by discipline.

ordering of items by difficulty level with more spread in difficulty when rated by physical therapists. This map shows stair climbing to be the most difficult item and wheelchair locomotion to be the easiest. The map also shows stair climbing to be rated more severely by physical therapists and wheelchair locomotion to be more severely rated by nurses. The item calibrations and fit statistics for each discipline are presented in Table 2, along with the item displacement for the anchored PT ratings. These results confirm the finding that stair climbing is rated less severely and wheelchair locomotion more severely by nurses. Again, because the sample is large, the standard errors for each item in each calibration are small, and minor differences that may not be clinically meaningful are statistically significant. Using the direct comparison across calibration values with a criterion of 0.08, the differences in difficulty level across disciplines are significant in all but one item; using item displacement with a criterion of 0.04, the cross-discipline ratings of all items are significantly different. Again, a more rigorous criterion is needed to distinguish clinically meaningful as opposed to statistically significant differences.

Table 2 also contains the fit statistics for each mobility item as rated by both sets of raters. These results show one item, wheelchair locomotion, to misfit for both disciplines (infit mean square of 1.58 for RN ratings and 2.29 for PT ratings) and another, stair climbing (infit mean square of 3.22) to misfit in the RN ratings, with the bed/chair/wheelchair transfer and toilet transfer items tending to overfit (infit mean square < 0.80) in the ratings of both disciplines and the walking and tub transfer items overfitting in the RN ratings. As with other analyses of these items, there is some duplication in the transfer items.[4,11]

Figure 5 presents the probability curve for the mobility items. Unlike the curves for the self-care items, these curves reveal different uses of the rating scale. The percentage of ratings in each category across disciplines presented in Table 3 indicates that physical therapists are less likely to use categories 2 and 3 (11% versus 25% for nurses) and more likely to use category 1 (25% versus 9% for nurses). A confounding factor is that a rating of 1 can mean either complete dependence or the item was not assessed.

Despite severity differences on individual items, average patient measures are only slightly higher when rated by nurses (0.07) than by physical therapists (–0.19). While the variability of RN ratings is greater (2.01 compared to 1.52 for PT ratings), the RMSE is also larger (0.69 compared to 0.52 for PT ratings); as a result, the person separation index is essentially the same for both (2.75 for RN ratings and 2.74 for PT ratings). Thus, while there are slight differences in average functional status when rated by nurses and physical therapists, the differentiation across functional status levels is essentially the same.

Figure 6 presents a plot of patient measures as rated by nurses and physical therapists for a subsample of patients rated by both. Because of the large sample size, the control lines are extremely narrow and many cases fall outside the 95% confidence area. As with the self-care items, the best fit line does not run parallel to the identity line; RN ratings are higher for patients with high functional levels and lower for patients with low functional levels. The net effect is that RN ratings of patient functional status are essentially the same as PT ratings. (The correlation between measures is 0.86.) This finding is confirmed by a *t*-test conducted on the means of the ratings by nurses and physical therapists for 4182 ratings; the average measure from the RN ratings (–0.32) is essentially the same as that from the PT ratings (–0.30) (*p*, NS).

RN Ratings on FIM Mobility Items:

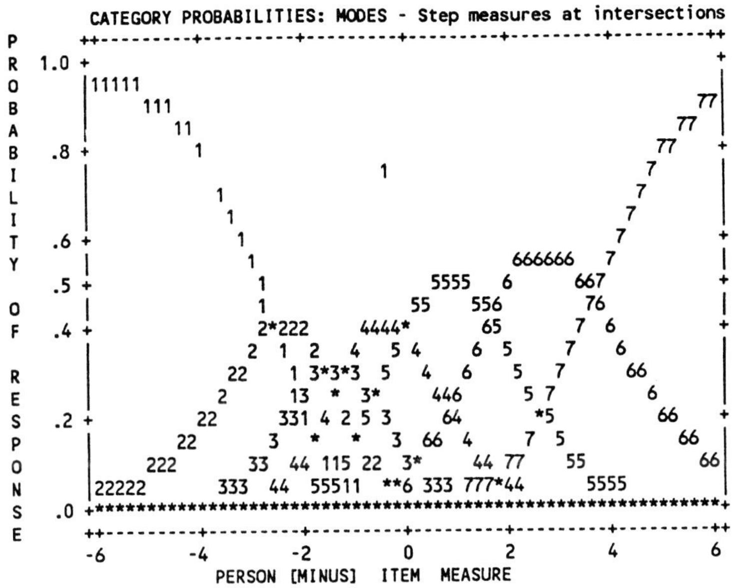

PT Ratings of FIM Mobility Items:

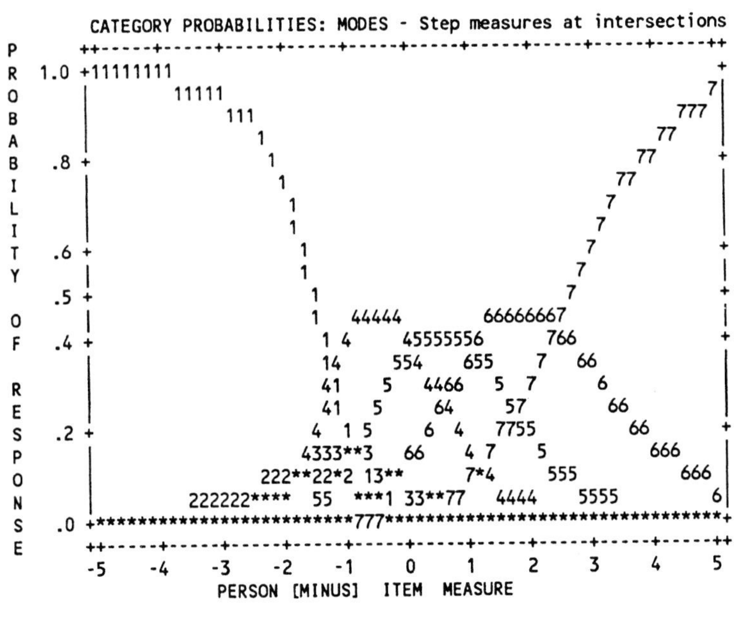

FIGURE 5. Probability curves for nurse and physical therapist ratings of mobility.

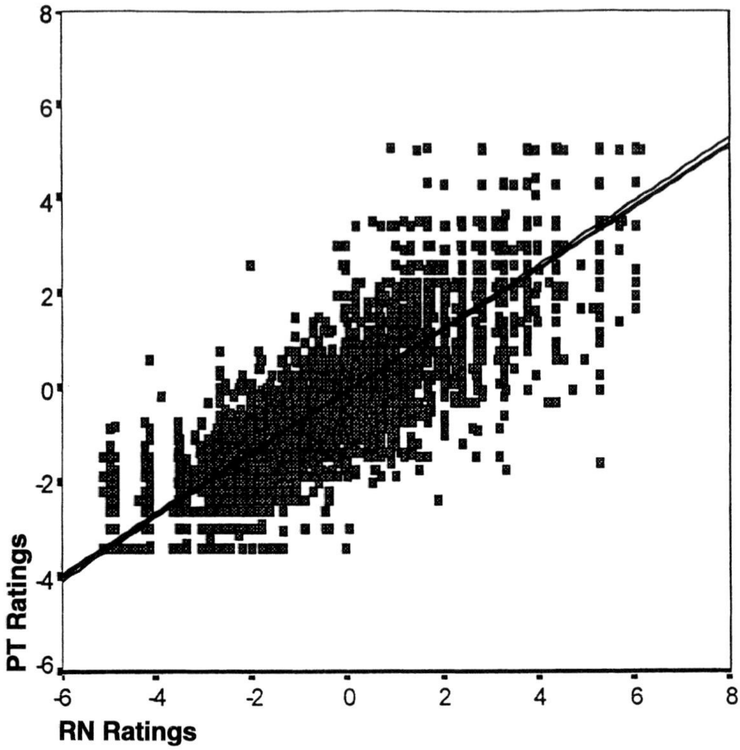

FIGURE 6. Person measures from nurse and physical therapist ratings of mobility. Note: Best fit curve +95% confidence intervals.

In summary, it appears that the difficulty level of mobility items are more spread out when rated by physical therapists, there is more misfit in the RN ratings, and the two disciplines use the rating categories differently for patients with lower functional status, perhaps because physical therapists do not assess lower-functioning patients as often. The average patient measures from the individual calibrations show functional status to be higher when rated by nurses. However, when averages are based only on patients rated by both disciplines, functional status in mobility is rated essentially the same by nurses and physical therapists.

Communication Items

The results of the calibrations of RN ratings and speech/language pathologist (SP) ratings show the variability in item calibrations to be greater for speech pathologists (0.98) than for nurses (0.42), with slightly more misfit in the SP ratings (infit mean square standard deviation of 0.35 for SP ratings and 0.10 for RN ratings). On the individual item level, the item map (Fig. 7) shows differences not only in the spread of item difficulty but also in the ordering of items by difficulty level. For nurses, vocal expression is the easiest item and visual comprehension is the most difficult; for speech pathologists, auditory comprehension is the easiest item and written expression is the most difficult. The items calibrations and fit statistics for each discipline are presented in Table 2, along with the item displacement for the

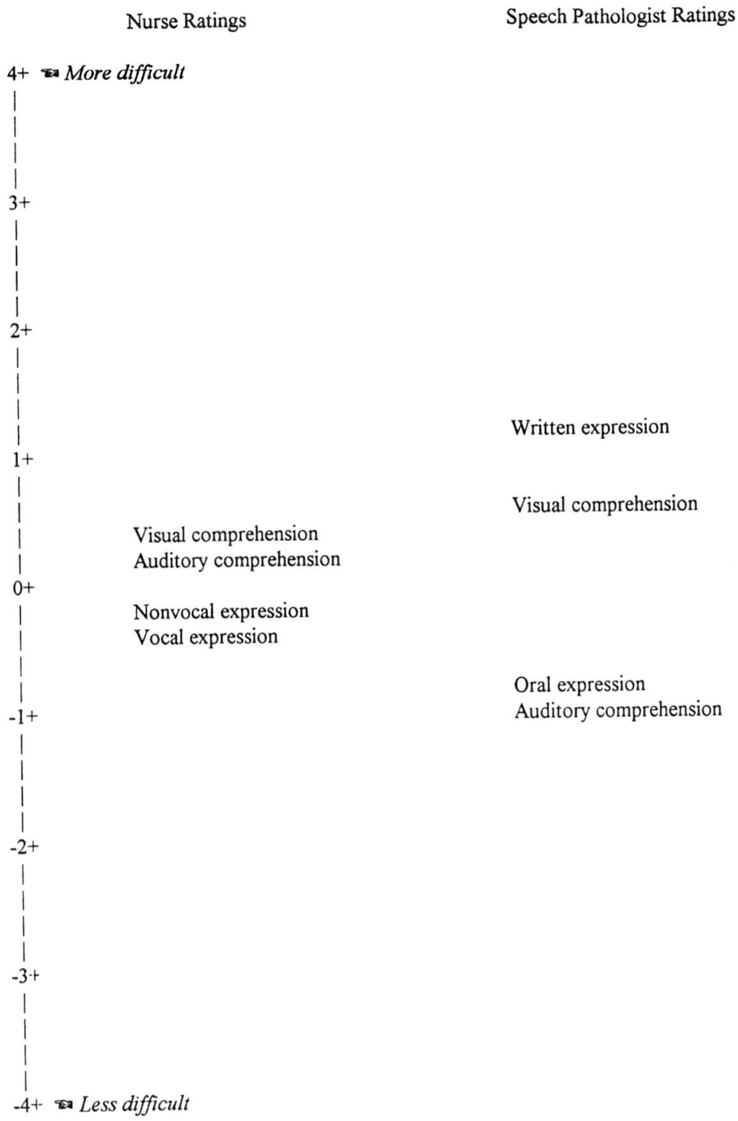

FIGURE 7. Communication item difficulties by discipline.

anchored SP ratings. These results indicate that nurses are more severe in rating auditory comprehension, and speech pathologists are more severe in rating written expression. Because the sample is large, the standard errors for each item are small; therefore, minor differences in item calibrations across disciplines may be statistically significant but not clinically meaningful. Using a criterion of item calibration plus and minus two standard errors and item displacement greater than twice the RMSE for the anchored calibrations identifies *all* the items as having discrepant cross-discipline ratings. As with the other sets of items, a more rigorous criterion is needed to identify truly discrepant ratings.

RN Ratings of FIM Communication Items:

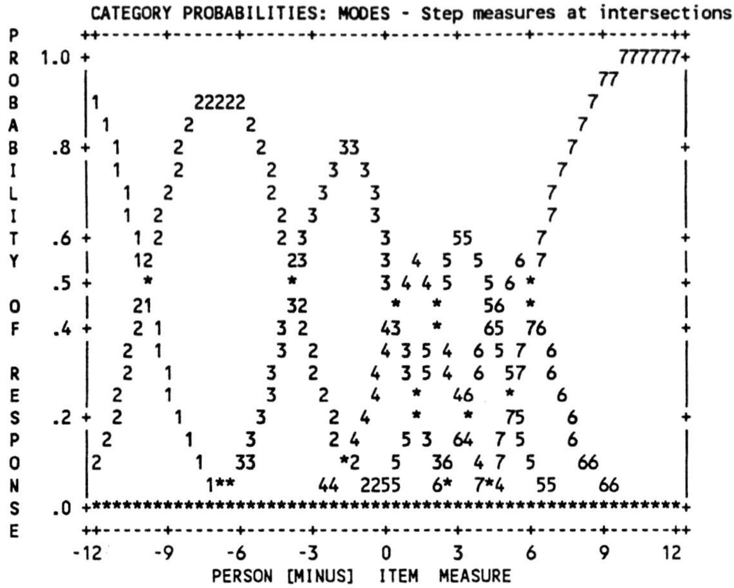

Speech Pathologist Ratings of FIM Communication Items:

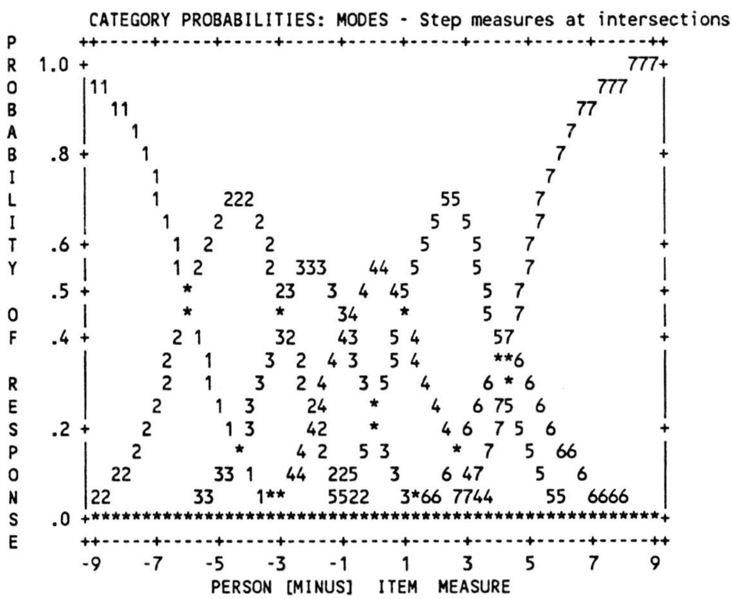

FIGURE 8. Probability curves for nurse and speech pathologist ratings of communication.

Table 2 also contains the fit statistics for each communication item as rated by both sets of raters. The results show one item, written expression, to misfit with the SP ratings (infit mean square = 1.61) and two others, oral expression and auditory comprehension, to slightly overfit the model (infit mean square < .80) for the SP ratings.

Figure 8 presents the probability curves for the RN and SP ratings of the communication items; these curves indicate that the two disciplines use the rating scale differently. Table 3 presents the percent of ratings at each rating scale category for both sets of raters; the results show that nurses are more likely to use categories 6 and 7 (33% versus 8% for speech pathologists) and speech pathologists are more likely to use categories 1 and 2 (34% versus 14% for nurses). A confounding factor is that in the RN ratings, a 1 may mean total assistance required or item not assessed, but in the SP ratings, a separate category, 0, exists for item not assessed.

The average person measures on the communication items as rated by speech pathologists were much lower (–1.43) than as rated by nurses (1.65). There was greater variability in the measures based on SP ratings (4.25 compared to 3.09 for the RN ratings) but the RMSE was also greater for speech pathologists (1.35 compared to 1.00 for nurses); as a result, the person separation index was essentially the same for both (2.99 for speech pathologists compared to 2.91 for nurses). Thus, patient functional status is lower when rated by speech pathologists, but their ratings differentiate across functional levels as well as those of nurses.

Figure 9 presents a plot of the patient measures on the communication items as rated by nurses and speech therapists for a subset of patients who were rated by both.

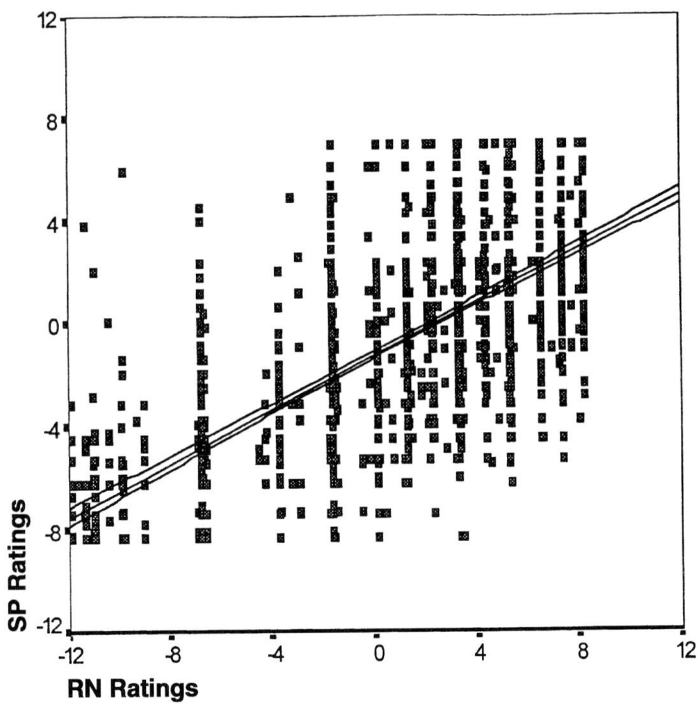

FIGURE 9. Person measures from nurse and speech pathologist ratings of communication. Note: Best fit curve +95% confidence intervals.

As with the other sets of items, because the sample is large and the standard error is small, the control lines are narrow and many cases fall outside the 95% confidence area. The best fit line does not run parallel to the identity line; RN ratings are higher for patients with high functional status and lower for patients with low functional status. The net effect is that speech pathologists are more severe raters in that the average person measures are higher when rated by nurses than when rated by speech pathologists. (The correlation between measures is 0.68.) This finding is confirmed by a t-test conducted on the means of the ratings by nurses and speech pathologists for 1819 ratings; the average measure from the RN ratings (1.02) was significantly higher and meaningfully different ($t = 19.2, p < .001$) than that from the SP ratings (–0.74).

In summary, it appears that speech pathologists rate communication items more severely; there is more misfit to the model in the SP ratings; nurses are more likely to rate patients as independent while speech pathologists are more likely to rate them as severely impaired; and the patient measures based on SP ratings are substantially lower than those from the RN ratings. The different rating scales used by RN and SP raters may explain these results.

DISCUSSION

A systematic bias in functional status ratings across disciplines would prevent meaningful comparisons of patient performance when different disciplines provided ratings. If the severity of ratings and the functional level of patients both vary, one cannot attribute differences in calibrations to rating severity alone. Thus, when the functional level of patients rated by one discipline is substantively different from the level of those rated by the other, the calibrations may differ systematically.

Functional status is rated by the disciplines from whom treatment is received. Physical and occupational therapy is provided to all patients. For this reason, one would not expect a difference between patients rated by nurses and those rated by occupational and physical therapists. Therefore, one would not expect a bias in the calibrations of the self-care and mobility items. However, this is ot the case for the communication items. Speech therapy is not provided to most patients; patients who receive speech therapy are more impaired in communication than those not receiving speech therapy. Thus, speech pathologists rate only more severely impaired patients on communication items while nurses rate all patients on these items. This difference could bias the results of the calibrations.

In this study the percentage of patients for whom both sets of ratings are available varied: self-care items = 73%; mobility items = 61%; communication items = 27%. To explore the possibility of a systematic difference in functional status of patients rated by one or both disciplines having an impact on item calibrations, two sets of items were recalibrated based only on patients who were rated by both disciplines: self-care and communication. For the self-care items, the differences were negligible in terms of severity of ratings; the RN and OT ratings were essentially the same whether the total sample or only patients who were rated by both disciplines were included in the sample. The patient ratings differed depending on which sample was used, but the differences were parallel for both disciplines; average functional status decreased when patients only rated by one discipline were deleted but the decrease was the same for both RN and OT ratings. Thus, while functional status level differed for the two samples, the item calibrations were the same regardless of the sample on which they were based, and both groups defined the construct similarly.

More differences were found in the item calibrations of the communication items; however, the differences were small and did not affect the ordering of items by difficulty. Restricting the sample only to patients rated by nurses and speech pathologists slightly spread out the difficulty levels based on the RN ratings and slightly decreased the spread in difficulty level based on the SP ratings. There was no effect on average person measures when rated by speech pathologists but there was a decrease when rated by nurses—as one would expect when less impaired patients are deleted from the sample. Thus, while functional status of the entire sample and the subsample differed, the item calibrations were affected minimally.

CONCLUSIONS

Several conclusions can be drawn based on these results. First, one needs to look at more than item difficulty when comparing the severity of ratings across disciplines; one also needs to examine item fit and use of the rating scale. Of the four items that misfit the model, two misfit in ratings by both disciplines and two misfit only in the ratings of one. High misfit by both disciplines would indicate a misfit of the items to the construct, but high misfit by only one discipline would indicate a rater problem. Therefore, if some items misfit only when rated by one discipline, it matters which discipline is doing the rating. Raters by discipline also differ in their use of the rating scale. Nurses and physical therapists differ in their use of the scale when rating patients with low functional status: physical therapists were more likely to rate patients as totally dependent while nurses were more likely to rate them as requiring moderate to maximal assistance. Nurses and speech pathologists also differ in their use of the rating scale. Nurses are more likely to rate patients as being independent in comprehension or expression, and speech pathologists are more likely to rate patients as severely or moderately severely impaired. The dual meaning of a rating of 1 and the use of different rating scales might also contribute to this result.

Second, more stringent criteria are needed to evaluate differences in item calibrations across disciplines and item displacement when anchoring is used. Using a criterion of two times the item standard errors or the RMSE identified all or almost all of the items as having significantly different difficulty levels across disciplines. The item maps, however, show large differences in only four items: wheelchair locomotion, stair climbing, auditory comprehension, and written expression. Using the standard error of the item mean or the person RMSE—while representing more stringent criteria—has no conceptual basis for this purpose.

Third, differences in results for all patients rated by either discipline versus patients rated by both disciplines are negligible, especially when dealing with large samples. Even in the case where data from both raters were available for less than 30% of the sample, the item calibrations and person measures varied little, lending confidence to the method used in this analysis. However, if systematic differences are a concern, the use of a procedure that does not require complete ratings of all subjects, such as FACETS, might be preferable.

REFERENCES

1. Elam JT, Graney MJ, Beaver T, et al: Comparison of subjective ratings of function with observed functional ability of frail older persons. Am J Public Health 81:1127–1130, 1991.
2. Hamilton BB, Granger CV, Sherwin SF, et al: A uniform national data system for medical rehabilitation. In Fuhrer MJ (ed): Rehabilitation Outcomes: Analysis and Measurement. Baltimore, Brooks, 1987.
3. Heinemann AW, Hamilton B, Linacre JM, et al: Functional status and therapeutic intensity during inpatient rehabilitation. Am J Phys Med Rehabil 74:315–326, 1995.
4. Heinemann AW, Hamilton BB, Wright BD, et al: Rating scale analysis of functional assessment measures. Final Report. National Institute on Disability and Rehabilitation Research, 1991.

5. Heinemann AW, Kirk P, Hastie BA, et al: Relationships between disability measures and nursing effort during medical rehabilitation for patients with traumatic brain and spinal cord injury. Arch Phys Med Rehabil 78:143–149, 1997.
6. Heinemann AW, Linacre JM, Wright BD, et al: Measurement characteristics of the Functional Independence Measure. Top Stroke Rehabil 1(3):1–15, 1994.
7. Heinemann AW, Linacre JM, Wright BD, et al: Prediction of rehabilitation outcomes with disability measures. Arch Phys Med Rehabil 75:133–143, 1994.
8. Jaworski DM, Kult T, Boynton PR: The Functional Independence Measure: A pilot study comparison of observed and reported ratings. Rehabil Nurs Res 3:141–147, 1994.
9. Kaufert JM: Functional ability indices: Measurement problems in assessing their validity. Arch Phys Med Rehabil 64:260–267, 1983.
10. Linacre JM: Item and step calibrations for Functional Independence Measure items [manuscript], 1991.
11. Linacre JM, Heinemann AW, Wright BD, et al: The structure and stability of the Functional Independence Measure. Arch Phys Med Rehabil 75:127–132, 1994.
12. Linacre JM, Heinemann AW, Wright BD, Granger CV: The Functional Independence Measure as a measure of disability. Chicago, Rehabilitation Services Evaluation Unit, Rehabilitation Institute of Chicago, 1991, research report 91-01.
13. Linacre JM, Wright BD: BIGSTEPS: Rasch Analysis for all Two-Facet Models. Chicago, MESA Press, 1996.
14. Myers AM, Holliday PJ, Harvey KA, Hutchinson KS: Functional performance measures: Are they superior to self-assessments? J Gerontol 48:M196–206, 1993.
15. Sorenson JB, Klee M, Palshof T, Hansen HH: Performance status assessment in cancer patients: An inter-observer variability study. Br J Cancer 67:773–775, 1993.
16. Valleron AJ, Vallery-Masson J, Poitrenaud J, Bourlier F: Health as felt by the subject and assessed by the physician: Methods for measurement and evaluation in a population of subjects in their sixties. Biomed Pharmacother 37:441–446, 1993.
17. Velozo CA, Pan AW, Magalhaes LC, Leiter P: Nurse-therapist differences in ADL assessment [abstract]. Arch Phys Med Rehabil 75:720, 1994.
18. Weinberger M, Samsa GP, Schmader K, et al: Comparing proxy and patients' perceptions of patients' functional status: Results from an outpatient geriatric clinic. J Am Geriatr Soc 40:585–588, 1992.
19. Wright BD, Linacre JM, Heinemann AW: Measuring functional status in rehabilitation. New Dev Funct Assess 4:475–491, 1993.

INDEX

Entries in **boldface type** indicate complete chapters.